When Hope Feels Lost:

A Complete Guide To Supporting Him Through Treatment

Jay Richard

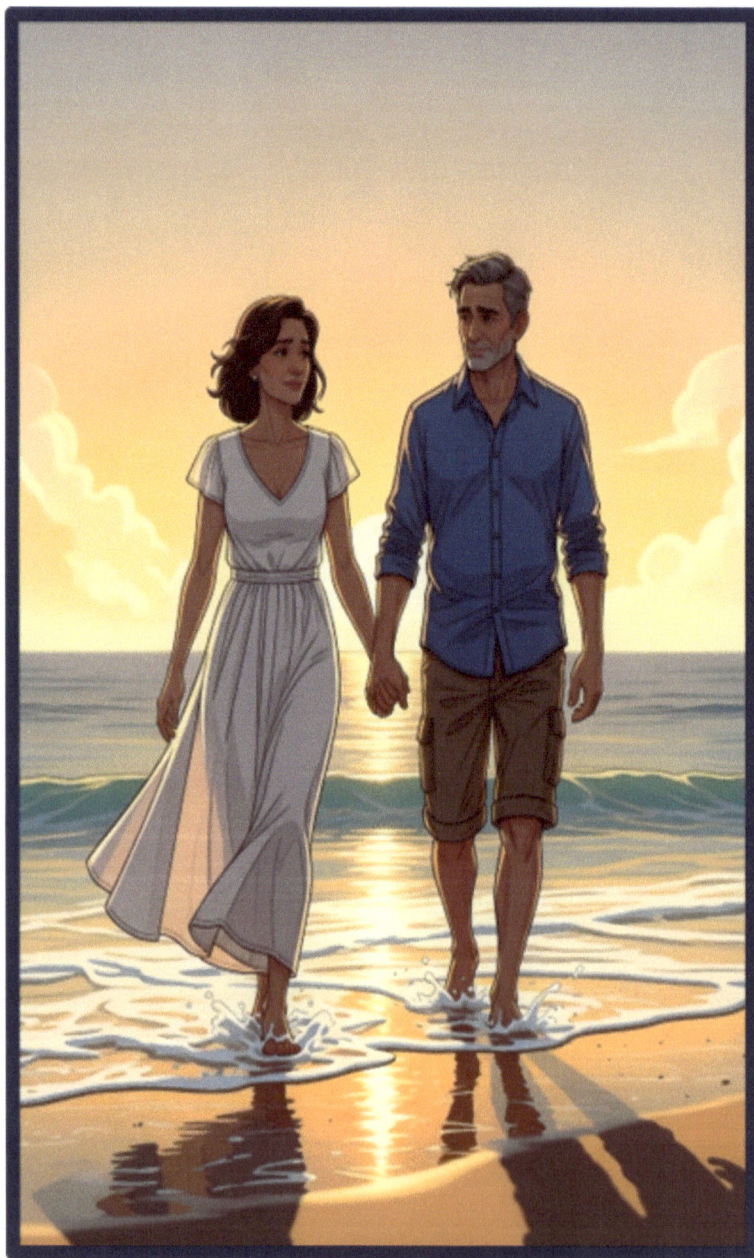

When Hope Feels Lost:

Copyright & Disclaimer

Content Warning: This book contains explicit discussions of sexual health, medical treatments, and clinical interventions related to erectile dysfunction. Content includes frank discussions of sexual function, intimate relationships, and medical procedures that some readers may find sensitive.

Medical Disclaimer: This book is intended solely for informational and educational purposes and should not be construed as medical advice or used as a substitute for professional medical consultation. The author is not a medical doctor and is not providing medical or therapeutic services through this publication. At times it may sound like the author is an expert or physician, but to be clear: he is not. The content represents personal opinions and information gathered from various sources, and all information should be independently verified.

Always consult with qualified healthcare providers, including urologists, primary care physicians, endocrinologists, or other specialists, before making any decisions regarding erectile dysfunction treatment, medication, or lifestyle changes. Individual circumstances vary significantly, and what may be appropriate for one person may not be suitable for another. Sexual health conditions can have complex underlying causes that require proper medical evaluation and diagnosis. If you are experiencing severe symptoms or have concerns about your sexual health, please consult with a healthcare professional promptly.

Limits of Liability: The author and publisher shall not be liable for misuse of this material. The author is specifically not giving medical or legal advice. All decisions are taken at your own risk. Get proper medical advice from doctors before making your decision.

For additional resources and updates: www.jayrichard.com

Foreword

When I wrote the foreword for Jay's first book about his journey with erectile dysfunction, I knew we were addressing a critical need: *helping men understand they are not alone in this struggle.* However, as I reflected on the countless patients I have treated over the years, I realized we were missing a crucial voice in this conversation: *the partners.*

Erectile dysfunction does not affect just the man experiencing it. It ripples through relationships, creating waves of confusion, frustration, rejection, and often silent suffering for partners who feel powerless to help the person they love. In my practice, I have seen relationships strain under the weight of unspoken fears, misplaced blame, and the gradual erosion of intimacy that ED can bring.

Partners often become the hidden casualties of this condition. They may question their attractiveness, wonder if they are somehow at fault, or feel rejected and unloved when physical intimacy becomes complicated or disappears entirely. Many suffer in silence, unsure how to broach the subject or offer support without causing further embarrassment or distress.

This book fills a vital gap in the resources available to those navigating ED as a couple. Jay provides an honest, practical guide that acknowledges the complex emotions and challenges partners face. This book offers strategies for communication, understanding, and maintaining connection during what can be one of the most challenging periods in a relationship.

What makes this book particularly valuable is its dual perspective, combining Jay's firsthand experience as someone who has successfully overcome ED with insights from the partner's viewpoint. This comprehensive approach provides couples with tools to not just survive this challenge, but to emerge stronger and more connected.

As healthcare providers, we often focus on the medical aspects of treatment, but healing extends far beyond the physical. Relationships require their own form of medicine: patience, understanding, open communication, and hope. This book provides that medicine.

To the partners reading this: your feelings are valid, your role is crucial, and your relationship can not only survive this challenge but thrive. You are not powerless in this journey, and you are certainly not alone.

May this book serve as your road map to navigating these difficult waters together, and may it remind you that with understanding, patience, and the right resources, love truly can conquer all obstacles.

By William Figlesthaler, M.D., FACS

Table of Contents

For information regarding bulk purchases,
educational use, or special editions,
please contact the publisher at: info@seibroinc.com

This book is a work of original authorship.
Author: Jay Richard
Layout, design, and typography by Seibro Inc.
Published by Seibro Inc
Tampa, FL

Printed in the United States of America
First Edition, 2025
JayRichard.com

10 9 8 7 6 5 4 3 2 1

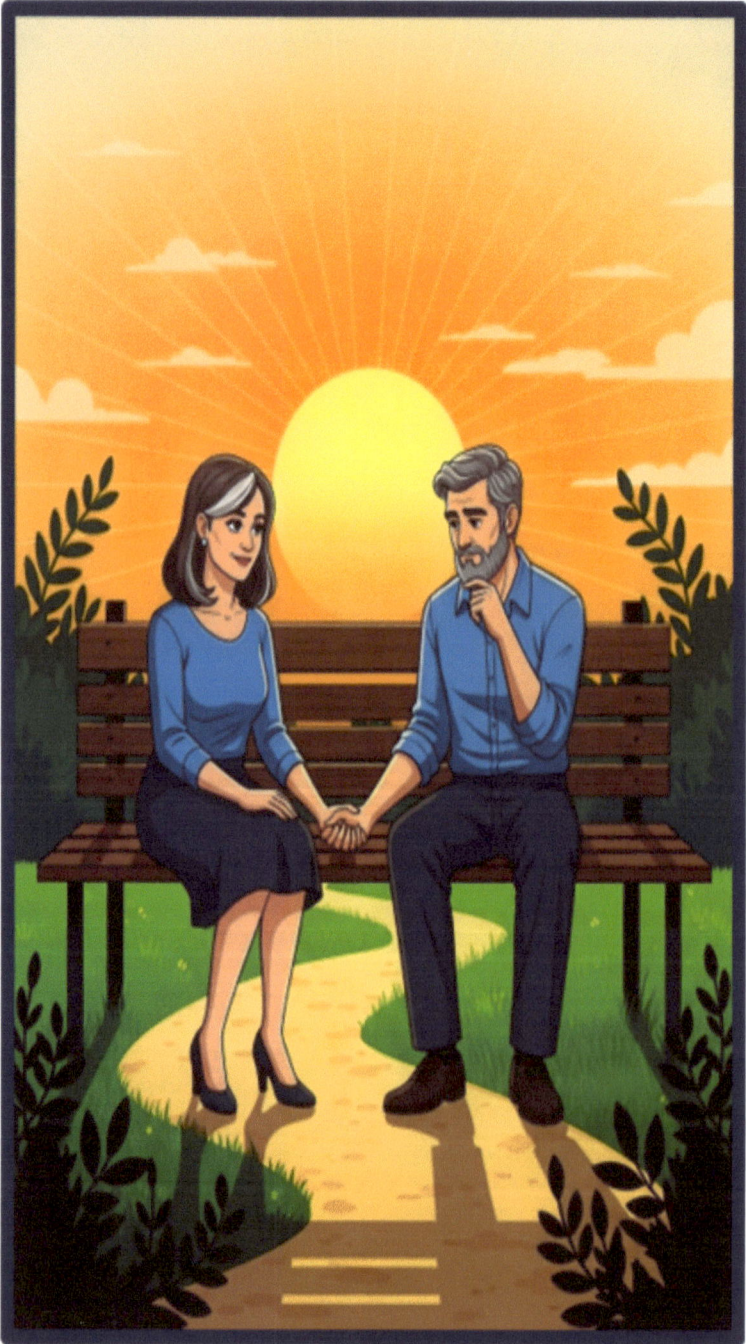

Author's Note

When I wrote my first book about erectile dysfunction, I shared my journey as someone facing this challenge while single. That experience taught me about the medical and emotional sides of ED, but it also showed me something crucial: the partners in our lives need their own voice in this conversation.

This book speaks from the perspective of someone in a committed relationship because that's what will help you most, the partner seeking guidance and hope. What you'll hear throughout these pages comes from all my experiences with ED, including insights that have shaped my understanding of what truly helps couples get through this together.

Everything in this book has been tested in real life, including my current long-term relationship where we've used many of these approaches successfully. More than that, it reflects what I've learned about the difference between couples who barely survive ED and those who come out stronger.

My goal is simple: to give you the most helpful guidance possible. The heart of partnership: supporting each other, talking honestly, and solving problems together. This stays the same whether you learn it through one relationship or many.

What you'll find here isn't theory. It's real experience from someone who has lived with ED and discovered, sometimes the hard way, what works. You deserve to feel less alone, better informed, and genuinely hopeful about what's ahead.

Jay Richard

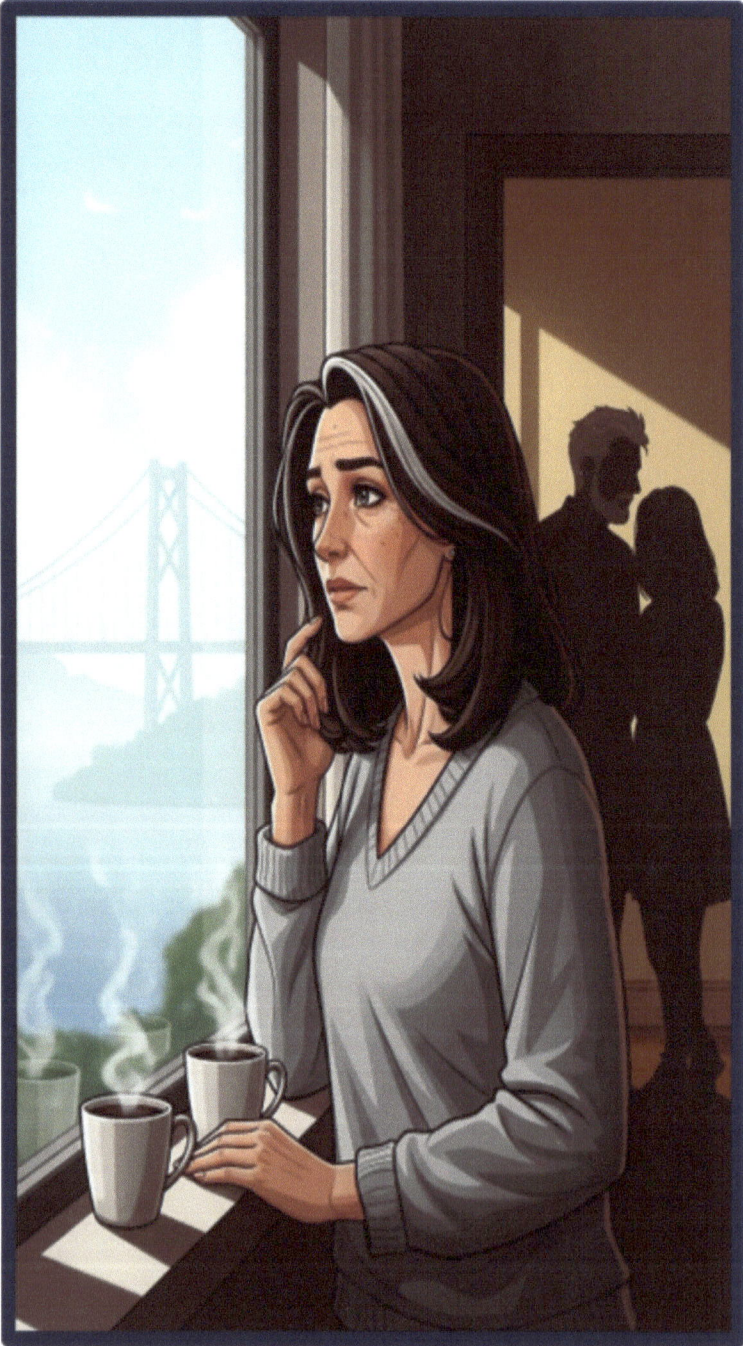

Introduction: The Hidden Journey

I'm writing this book for you, the woman standing beside a man struggling with ED. If you're confused, hurt, or somehow think you are responsible for what's happening, I want you to know something important right from the start: this has nothing to do with anything you've done or failed to do.

When ED entered our relationship, I watched my partner try to navigate an experience no one discusses openly. While everyone focused on *my* body, *my* treatments, and *my* recovery, she was left trying to figure out this new reality on her own. She couldn't express her needs without seeming unsupportive. Her experience became invisible, even though she was just as affected by what both of us were going through.

After writing my first book about ED (*When Pills Stop Working*), which included a chapter on partners, I received a number of messages from women saying, *"This is exactly what I'm experiencing, but I need more. I need a guide written specifically for me."* They all expressed the same frustration: *"Everyone focuses on him,* but I'm struggling too, and I don't know how to help either of us."

Why This Book Exists

When ED shows up in a relationship, it affects both people equally, just differently. Partners face their own crisis while trying to provide support, often without understanding what's happening or what kind of help matters. You need your own road map, not just advice on how to support someone else.

This book exists because your experience matters. Your emotions are valid, your needs are important, and your role in recovery is crucial. You deserve guidance that acknowledges what you're going through while giving you practical tools to navigate this without losing yourself.

More than that, you deserve to know that couples don't just survive ED, but they often build stronger relationships because of what they learn while facing this together.

What You'll Discover

This isn't a medical textbook or generic relationship advice. It's a conversation between someone who's been there and someone who needs to know she's not crazy, not selfish, and not alone.

You'll realize that your uncertainty makes perfect sense-millions of women experience the same thing. You'll learn specific ways to discuss this difficult topic and discover what genuine support looks like versus what seems helpful but creates pressure.

Most importantly, you'll see concrete evidence that what you're facing now can become the foundation for deeper intimacy and stronger partnership than you've ever experienced.

You'll learn how to take care of yourself while supporting him, not because self-care is trendy, but because neglecting your own well-being helps no one. You'll discover how to express your needs without creating pressure and how to maintain hope when progress seems slow.

Your Path Forward

The road ahead may seem uncertain right now, but you don't have to walk it alone. Millions of couples have traveled this path successfully, and the strategies in this book come from real experience including both the failures that taught hard lessons and the breakthroughs that changed everything.

Your love story didn't end when ED began. It's evolving into something more resilient and consciously chosen than what you started with. The partnership you're creating through this experience will serve you for a lifetime.

Let's walk this path together.

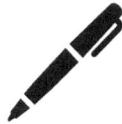

"Hope isn't pretending everything is fine;
it's believing the story isn't over yet."

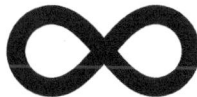

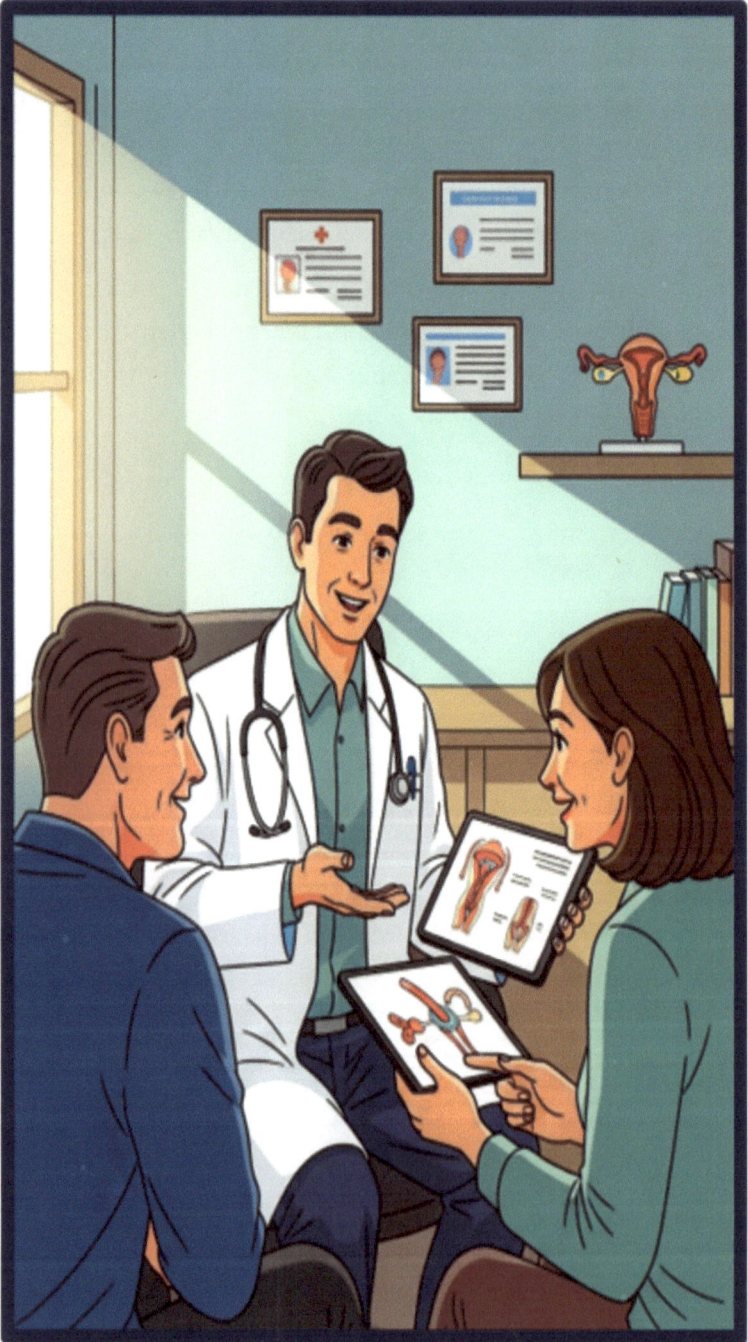

Chapter 1: Understanding ED

Let me start by telling you what I wish someone had explained to my partner when both of us were scared and confused about what was happening to my body. Understanding what ED really is, and what it isn't, became the first step in freeing both of us from thinking this was somehow about our relationship or her desirability.

The Most Important Thing You Need to Know

Before anything else, I need to address something that torments nearly every partner facing this situation: the belief that this is somehow about them. It's not.

It has nothing to do with your attractiveness, your sexual skills, or your desirability. His body's struggle doesn't reflect anything about you or what you bring to the relationship.

During my worst months with ED, I was more attracted to my partner than I'd ever been. My desperate desire for her and my body's ability to respond had become completely disconnected systems. Understanding that attraction and erectile function operate independently helped both of us stop taking this personally.

What Is Erectile Dysfunction

When my doctor first explained ED to me, he said it meant my body couldn't get hard or stay hard reliably during sex. That word *"reliably"* struck me most. This wasn't about the occasional off night when stress or exhaustion affected things. This was about my body consistently failing to cooperate, no matter how much I wanted her.

You're Not Alone

About 30 million men in the United States struggle with ED. By 40, almost half of all men deal with this. Learning these numbers helped my partner realize we weren't some rare, broken case. Suddenly, she understood that millions of other women were probably experiencing exactly what she was going through.

How Things Actually Work (It's More Complicated Than You Think)

I used to think erections were simple, like flipping a light switch. But my doctor helped me understand it's more like starting an old car on a cold morning-everything has to work together perfectly. When even one part isn't cooperating, the whole thing falls apart:

- **The brain connection:** Performance anxiety became the noise that drowned out the delicate communication between my brain and body. Even when I desperately wanted her, my worried mind would interfere with the signals my body needed.

- **The physical systems:** Blood vessels need to open up and close off in perfect coordination. Heart disease, diabetes, or high blood pressure can interfere with this process. I learned that the same circulation problems that affect your heart also affect erections.

- **The hormone factor:** Testosterone and other hormones need to be balanced. Thyroid problems or other hormonal imbalances can throw everything off. Even stress hormones can shut down the whole system.

- **The mental component:** Your mental state-stress levels, confidence, anxiety, depression-influences every other system. This was perhaps the most difficult part for my partner to understand initially. How could psychological factors affect something as physical as an erection? But I learned that stress hormones literally restrict blood flow to the exact places you need it most.

When any one of these systems isn't working properly, erections become unreliable or impossible, regardless of attraction, desire, or relationship quality.

What Really Causes ED

Understanding the real causes was crucial for my partner's healing process. When she realized that none of these causes were related to her, she could stop analyzing our relationship for problems that didn't exist.

- **The physical stuff** that can cause ED surprised me: heart problems, diabetes, blood pressure issues, and tons of common medications including the blood thinner I was taking. Even allergy pills can mess things up. Smoking, drinking too much, being significantly overweight, or injuries and surgeries can all contribute.

- **Psychological causes** include depression, anxiety, work stress, financial pressure, family problems, performance anxiety, or past trauma. What shocked me was learning that stress about anything-not just sexual performance-can trigger ED.

- **Lifestyle factors** include lack of exercise, poor diet, inadequate sleep, or chronic stress from any source. I realized my poor sleep and high-stress job were probably contributing more than I'd thought.

Learning that ED could be caused by everything from blood pressure medication to work stress helped her understand that this truly had nothing to do with her or us as a couple.

Myths That Make Everything Worse

These myths were causing her much unnecessary pain:

- **"If he's attracted to me, he should be able to get an erection."** This myth nearly destroyed her self-esteem. The reality is that my desperate attraction to her and my body's ability to respond were separate systems that had stopped communicating. It's like having a car with a full tank of gas but a broken starter. The fuel is there, but the engine won't turn over.

- **"ED means he's not interested in sex anymore"** She started believing my avoidance meant I had lost interest entirely. The reality was the opposite. I wanted intimacy desperately but was terrified of another failure. My withdrawal was about protecting myself from shame, not about losing desire for her.

- **"If we just communicate better, the ED will go away."** Good communication is essential for support, but it's not a medical cure. Communication helped us work as a team, but it couldn't fix blood flow problems or medication side effects. Love doesn't cure medical conditions, though it certainly helps you navigate them together.

There Is Real Hope

When I started researching treatment possibilities, I was amazed by how many effective solutions existed. Lifestyle changes can make a significant difference. Pills help about 6-7 out of 10 men. Injection therapy, vacuum devices, and penile implants offer other paths forward-with implants, 9 out of 10 couples report high satisfaction.

The key insight for both of us was this: treatment success isn't just about sexual performance; it's about rebuilding a satisfying intimate relationship together. With today's options, there's genuine reason for hope.

When she first learned about these treatment possibilities, she had concrete hope for the first time since my problems started. Instead of feeling helpless, both of us felt empowered. We weren't victims of this condition-we were partners working together toward a solution.

Most importantly, I learned that ED doesn't have to define our relationship or my identity as a man. It's a medical challenge that affects millions of couples, and like other medical challenges, it can be addressed with the right approach, patience, and support.

"ED may silence the body, but it doesn't silence the soul of a relationship unless you let it."

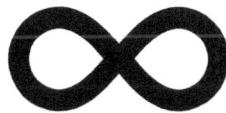

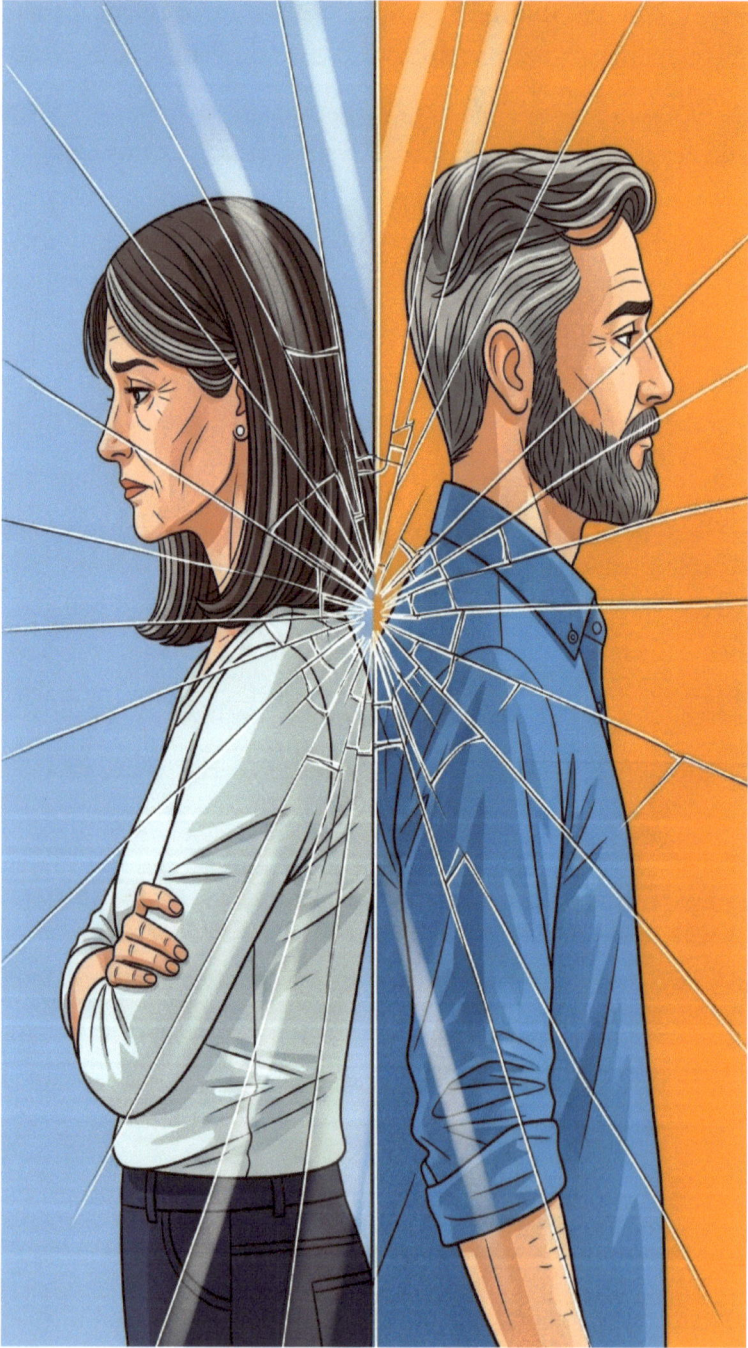

Chapter 2: Understanding Your Emotional Journey

As I said earlier, ED doesn't just happen to him. It happens to both of you. The emotional fallout is real. You are not alone. Women I've spoken with describe the same roller coaster of emotions. Once you understand the pattern, you can stop being blindsided and start navigating this together.

What You May Be Experiencing

Shock and Confusion

At first, it doesn't seem real. One woman described it as *"the ground shifting underneath me."* You were enjoying intimacy, building a life together, then suddenly asking yourself: *"how could this be happening?"* This disbelief is often the first reaction, and it's completely normal.

Your brain is trying to protect you from taking in too much at once. It's like a circuit breaker that trips when there's too much emotional voltage. Once that protective numbness starts to fade, your mind goes into detective mode, desperately trying to make sense of what's happening. That's when the self-doubt creeps in. Quietly at first, then with devastating force.

Self-Blame

Even knowing ED is medical, many women can't stop wondering, *"Is it me?"* My partner replayed our last intimate moments, searching for what she had done wrong. She tried new workouts, new approaches, convinced she could *"fix"* the problem if she became more attractive or skilled. Watching her carry that burden was almost heartbreaking because ED was never about her.

ED is a plumbing and wiring problem in his body, not a reflection of how he appreciates you. When a man can't get an erection, it's usually because blood isn't flowing right, nerves aren't firing properly, or hormones are out of whack.

Most of the time, ED comes from stuff happening inside his body, not between the two of you. Diabetes messes with blood flow. Heart problems affect circulation everywhere, including there. Even blood pressure medication can shut things down. His body isn't rejecting you-it's struggling with internal systems that aren't working properly.

Even as she intellectually understood my body was struggling with medical issues, her heart couldn't escape being hurt. Every failed intimate moment left her wondering if she was somehow being turned away.

The Rejection That Cuts Deep

Logically, you know your partner wants you. Emotionally, it seems like his body is saying no. That's a wound that cuts deep. She told me it was like abandonment.

Your heart knows the truth, but your gut doesn't believe it yet. The part of your brain that handles emotions is separate from the part that handles logic. When his body can't respond, your emotional brain screams *"rejection!"* even while you're thinking brain whispers *"medical condition."* It's not weakness. It's how we're wired. Your emotions make perfect sense, even when they don't match the facts.

That sense of rejection gradually transforms into something else: a desperate need to do something, anything, to fix what seems broken between you.

Frustration and Helplessness

Partners often become researchers, frantically searching the internet for supplements, diets, treatments. Her heart was in the right place, but every *"solution"* she presented only reminded me I was broken. Her helplessness turned into pressure for both of us.

I call this the *"fixer's trap."* When someone you love is hurting, every instinct tells you to solve it. But the more solutions you offer, the more pressure you accidentally create. Every supplement suggestion, every article you share, every gentle *"have you tried..."* reminds him that something's wrong with his body. Your love turns into pressure, and pressure is kryptonite for erections.

When all her efforts to research and solve our problem didn't create the breakthrough she hoped for, something shifted. The frantic energy gave way to a deeper sadness she hadn't expected.

Grief

Many women don't realize they're grieving, but that's exactly what it is: grieving the spontaneous intimacy you once had, the confidence you saw in him, the future you imagined together. Acknowledging this loss isn't weakness. It's honesty.

What you're experiencing has stages, just like any other loss:

- First comes denial: *"This is just temporary stress."*
- Then anger: *"This isn't fair to either of us."*

- Next is bargaining: *"If I just lose ten pounds, it'll get better."*

- Then sadness: *"Nothing will ever be spontaneous again."*

- And finally, acceptance: *"The two of us can figure this out together."*

Knowing these stages exist helps you realize that what seems chaotic, and overwhelming follows a predictable path. You're not losing your mind. You're grieving.

What He May Be Going Through

While you're wrestling with self-doubt, your partner is fighting his own battle. Let me share what was happening in my head during those months, because understanding this helped my partner realize both of us were struggling, just in different ways.

The Shame That Swallowed Me Whole

I'll never forget the first time I couldn't get an erection. I lay there afterward, staring at the ceiling, convinced I'd just lost my membership card to being a man. It sounds dramatic, but that's honestly how it was.

Shame doesn't just hurt emotionally. It hurts physically.

When a man can't get an erection, his brain processes it like a physical injury. The same part of your brain that screams when you break a bone also screams when your masculinity is broken. When I say it was like being punched in the gut, that's not just a metaphor. My brain was literally treating ED like trauma.

The next morning, I couldn't look her in the eye while she made coffee. Every time she smiled at me, I thought she was just being kind to the broken guy she was stuck with. When she reached for my hand, I pulled away. Not because I didn't want her touch, but because I didn't think I deserved it.

That shame became my constant companion. It whispered to me during work meetings: *"Everyone here can perform except you."* It followed me to the gym: *"All these guys are real men."* It even ruined watching movies together because any romantic scene reminded me of what I couldn't do anymore.

When Intimacy Became My Enemy

After the third time my body betrayed me, something changed. Instead of looking forward to being close with her, I started dreading it. Every kiss became the beginning of a test I was going to fail. Every loving touch became pressure.

Performance anxiety is twisted logic: your brain, trying to protect you from future *"failure,"* creates stress that makes failure inevitable. When you're anxious, your body basically cuts off blood flow to the exact places you need it most. It's like your brain is trying to save you from drowning by cutting off your air supply. Fear of ED becomes the very thing that causes ED.

I started going to bed later than her, hoping she'd be asleep. I'd work late, pick fights about silly things, anything to avoid the possibility of intimacy. I told myself I was protecting both of us from disappointment, but really, I was just scared.

The irony? I wanted her more than ever. I'd watch her getting ready in the morning and ache with longing, but my body had become this unpredictable stranger I couldn't trust. It was like being hungry but afraid to eat because the food might poison you.

The Fear That Kept Me Awake

My biggest terror wasn't about sex. It was about losing her. I'd lie awake creating horror stories in my head:

- *"She's going to realize she's too young for this."*

- *"She's going to find someone whose body actually works."*

- *"She's going to leave and tell everyone what's wrong with me."*

When you're already vulnerable, your brain becomes like an overprotective security guard, seeing threats everywhere. My mind would take any normal relationship moment and spin it into proof that she was going to leave. Patient smile? She's just being nice until she finds someone better. Gentle touch? She's saying goodbye. My brain's alarm system got stuck in the "on" position, flooding my body with stress chemicals that made everything worse.

Why I Pulled Away

The part that probably hurt her most, and it took me months to understand what I was doing. I started withdrawing from all kinds of affection-not just sexual, but everything. I stopped reaching for her hand. I gave quick, distracted hugs. I avoided long eye contact.

Men think they're being considerate when they pull away, but they're creating the exact problem they're trying to avoid. I thought I was protecting her from disappointment, but I was just protecting myself from another failure.

In my twisted logic, I thought I was being considerate. "If I don't show affection, she won't expect it to lead anywhere, and then both of us won't have to face another disappointment." I was trying to protect both of us, but I ended up making her feel rejected and unloved.

I didn't realize that by avoiding all intimacy, I was creating exactly what I feared most: distance between us. The ED wasn't pushing her away. My response to it was.

The Downward Spiral

All these emotions fed off each other like some kind of emotional tornado. Each one picked up the next until I was caught in this spinning mess that fed on itself. The shame made me anxious about performance, which made me withdraw, which made me a failure as a partner, which increased my fear of losing her, which made the shame even worse. It's like being caught in emotional quicksand. The more you struggle, the deeper you sink.

Some mornings I'd wake up and think, "Maybe today will be different." But by evening, after a day of carrying all this weight around, I'd be convinced nothing would ever be normal again. It was like being trapped in a room where the walls kept closing in.

What I Wish I'd Known Then

Looking back, I realize I was drowning in stories I'd made up about what ED meant about me as a man and as a partner. I thought it meant I was broken, that I was failing her, that our relationship was doomed.

The game-changer for me was finally believing that ED isn't a character flaw-*it's a medical problem*. When you understand that your body is malfunctioning, rather than your manhood failing, everything shifts. Men who get that ED is *"plumbing, not personality,"* recover faster and keep better relationships while they're figuring it out.

What I couldn't see then was that my partner wasn't judging my masculinity by my erections. She wasn't keeping score of sexual successes and failures. She just wanted both of us to figure it out together.

The hardest part for her wasn't the ED itself. It was watching *me* disappear emotionally while she had no idea how to help. *She needed her partner back, challenges and all.*

Moving Forward Together

Recognizing these patterns in ourselves was the first step toward healing. Once both of us understood that our emotional responses were completely normal, we could start figuring out what we needed from each other.

What you need:

- •Space to process without being judged.

- •Reassurance of his attraction.

- •Affection without sexual pressure.

- •Support outside the relationship.

What he needs:

- •Unconditional love not tied to performance.

- •Patience with his ups and downs.

- •Respect for his autonomy in seeking treatment.

- •Emotional safety to express his worries.

Right now, it may seem like chaos, but these emotions won't last forever. Most couples move from shock and loss into adjustment and even growth. The key is separating ED from your worth and from the core of your relationship.

You can't cure ED yourself, but you can decide how to walk through it together. With patience, communication, and perspective, this difficult season can become a foundation for deeper love and resilience.

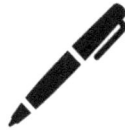

"Your worth is never defined by performance,
it's revealed in how you love, listen, and
show up for each other."

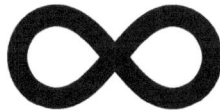

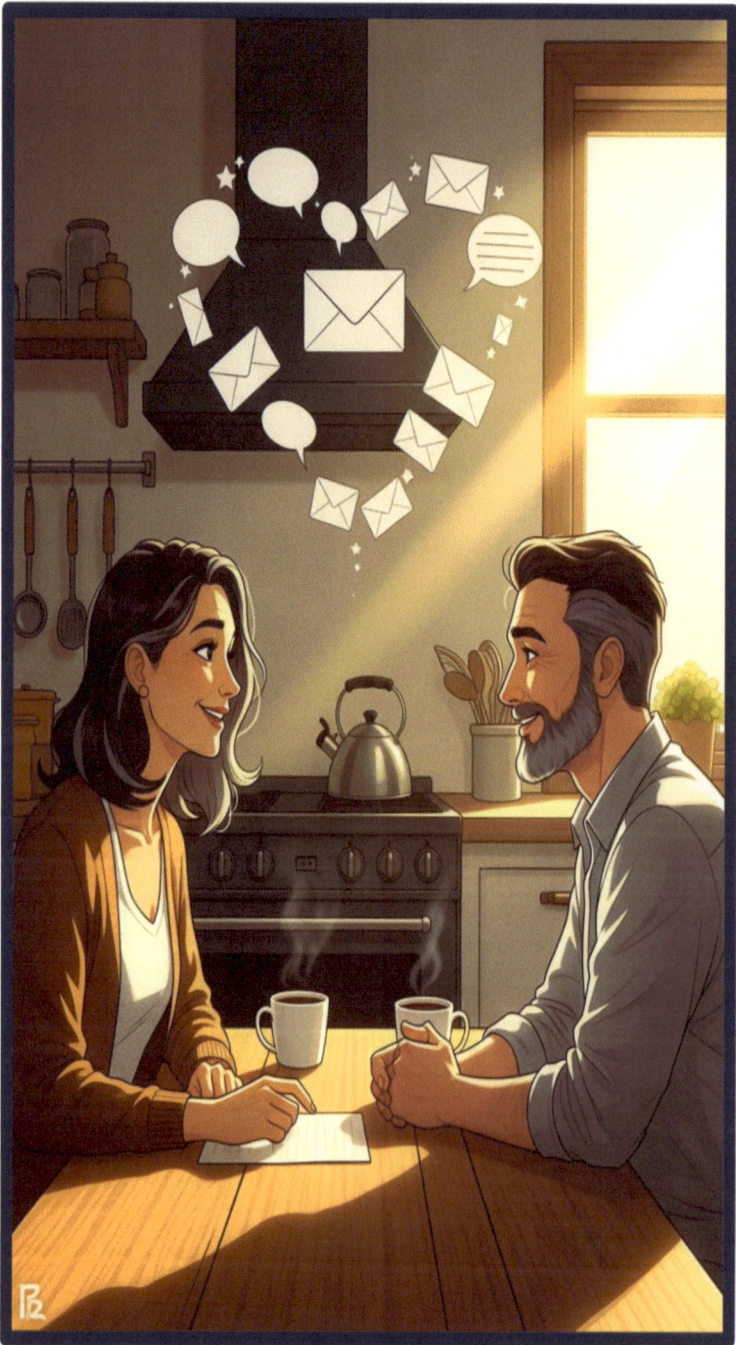

Chapter 3: Learning to Talk Again

ED didn't just disrupt our sex life. It disrupted our ability to communicate with each other.

Those intense emotions both of us had been carrying created an invisible wall between us. Topics that used to flow naturally suddenly became emotional landmines. But learning to communicate about this impossible subject? That became our lifeline.

When Words Become Impossible

Both of us became experts at avoiding the topic. There we were, facing the biggest challenge of our relationship, and neither of us could literally say "ED" or "erectile dysfunction" out loud.

I'll never forget lying in bed after another failed attempt. I wanted to say something, anything, to acknowledge what had just happened. But the shame was burning so hot in my chest that words felt impossible. She wanted to comfort me but was terrified of making me feel worse.

So, neither of us said anything. Both of us would roll over, turn away from each other, and pretend to sleep while our minds raced with everything neither of us could say.

The reasons for our silence ran deep:

- I thought discussing ED would make it more real and devastating.
- She feared expressing her needs would pressure me.

- Neither of us knew what words to use.

- Medical terms felt cold, euphemisms felt juvenile.

- My need for processing time felt like withdrawal to her.

- Her need to communicate felt like pressure to me.

We were stuck.

My First Attempt at "The Talk" (And Why It Failed)

I picked the worst possible moment. Bedtime, after a stressful day, in our bedroom. I was secretly hoping both of us could discuss it and then fix everything with perfect sex.

I basically ambushed her. Without warning, I announced that both of us needed to discuss my problem while she was getting ready for bed.

Her face immediately showed panic. She asked what she'd done wrong.

I fumbled around, trying to reference my issue without naming it. I couldn't even say "erectile dysfunction."

The words came out accusatory and desperate. Within ten minutes, both of us were near tears, both defensive, both more hurt than when the conversation started. I ended up sleeping on the couch.

Everything about that conversation was wrong. The moment I chose was terrible. I gave no warning or context. My language was vague and blame focused. Worst of all, I expected immediate resolution.

Our Communication Breakthrough

Our breakthrough came the next Sunday morning on our back patio with coffee. Neither of us planned what happened next.

That conversation taught us what both of us needed for future discussions.

Without really thinking, I apologized for how difficult this was on her. Instead of defensiveness, she just looked sad. She said she didn't need an apology; she just missed me. Not just sexually. She missed being close to me in all the ways both of us used to be connected.

I told her I missed her too. I missed being myself with her.

That conversation lasted two hours. For the first time, both of us were honest about our experience without trying to protect each other from painful truths. Neither of us was trying to fix anything. Both of us were just trying to understand each other.

What Finally Worked for Both of Us

Creating the Right Environment

Safe moments and settings became crucial. Weekend mornings worked best when both of us were rested, unhurried, emotionally available. Our back patio became sacred space where both of us could focus entirely on each other.

Starting with Love, Not Problems

Instead of announcing that both of us needed to discuss my problem, I learned to lead with care. I'd say things like how much I loved her and wanted to make sure both of us were supported or acknowledge that this was tough to discuss but I cared too much to keep pretending everything was fine.

Discussing Emotions, Not Just Facts

Before either of us could solve anything, both of us needed to understand how ED was affecting each of us emotionally.

Learning to share what was really happening inside became essential for me. I had to express how ashamed I felt when my body didn't cooperate, how that shame made me want to avoid her entirely, how I worried she'd get tired of this, how I missed being confident with her.

For her, expressing her real experience meant sharing how rejected she sometimes felt when intimacy didn't work out, even though she knew it wasn't about her. She needed to tell me how she missed our spontaneous connection and how she needed reassurance that I still desired her.

How You Can Lead Communication

You don't have to wait for him to bring it up. The silence is often worse than discussing it. Try gentle approaches like telling him you can see he's struggling and you're there for him or acknowledging that both of you have been distant and whatever you're dealing with, you're dealing with it together.

When he gets defensive, pause and address it with empathy rather than arguing. You might say; you can hear that felt like criticism, that wasn't your intention, that you think he's handling this with incredible courage, and ask if you can try saying it differently.

When you become overwhelmed, it's okay to take breaks. You can acknowledge that this brings up intense emotions for both of you and suggest coming back when you're more settled.

Be specific about what you need rather than hoping he'll guess. Tell him you miss being physically close and ask if both of you can find ways to stay connected. Let him know you need reminders that he still desires you and ask if he'd tell you what he loves about your body.

Conversation Starters That Worked for Us

For emotional check-ins: I learned to ask how she was doing about everything lately, not just the medical stuff, but how she was doing emotionally.

For treatment discussions: She would tell me she'd love to understand my treatment options, not to make decisions, but to be an informed support person, and ask how she could best help.

For addressing distance: One of us would say we missed being close and ask if both of us could discuss ways to stay connected while working through this.

The Power of Validation

This became our secret weapon. Instead of trying to fix each others emotions, both of us learned to acknowledge them. Validation doesn't mean agreement-it means understanding. It helps emotions pass more quickly because people truly hear each other.

When he expresses shame, instead of telling him he shouldn't experience that, try acknowledging that it makes complete sense he'd have those emotions when his body isn't cooperating.

When you experience rejection, instead of suppressing it, share it honestly. Let him know that while you understand this isn't personal, sometimes you still experience rejection when intimacy doesn't work out.

Your Communication Future

The skills both of us developed navigating ED now serve our relationship everywhere. Both of us can discuss any challenging topic with love and respect. Both of us learned to combine honesty with empathy.

Long after sexual function was restored, both of us continue benefiting from these communication tools. Your breakthrough moment is coming. This will happen when you realize you're not just discussing ED anymore. You are communicating with each other more honestly than ever before.

"The measure of a relationship isn't in perfect moments, but in the courage to stay when everything feels imperfect."

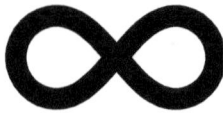

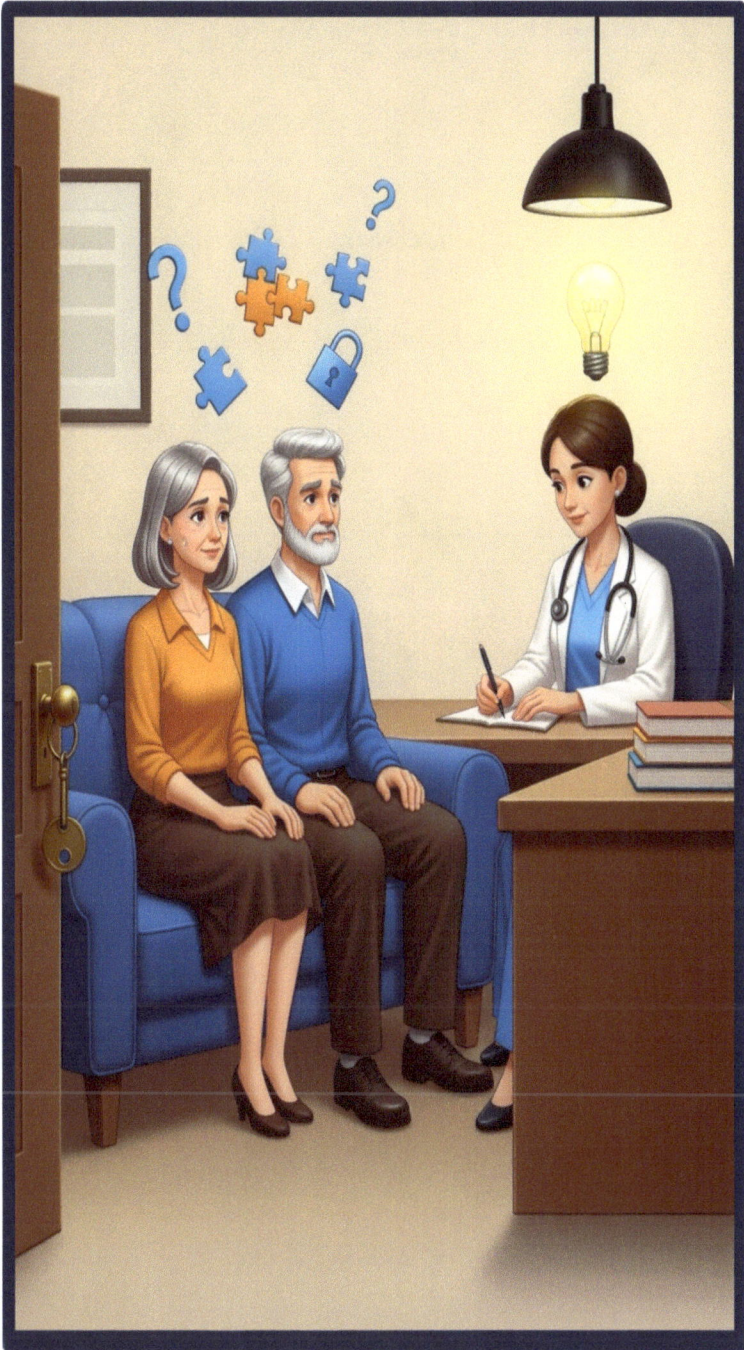

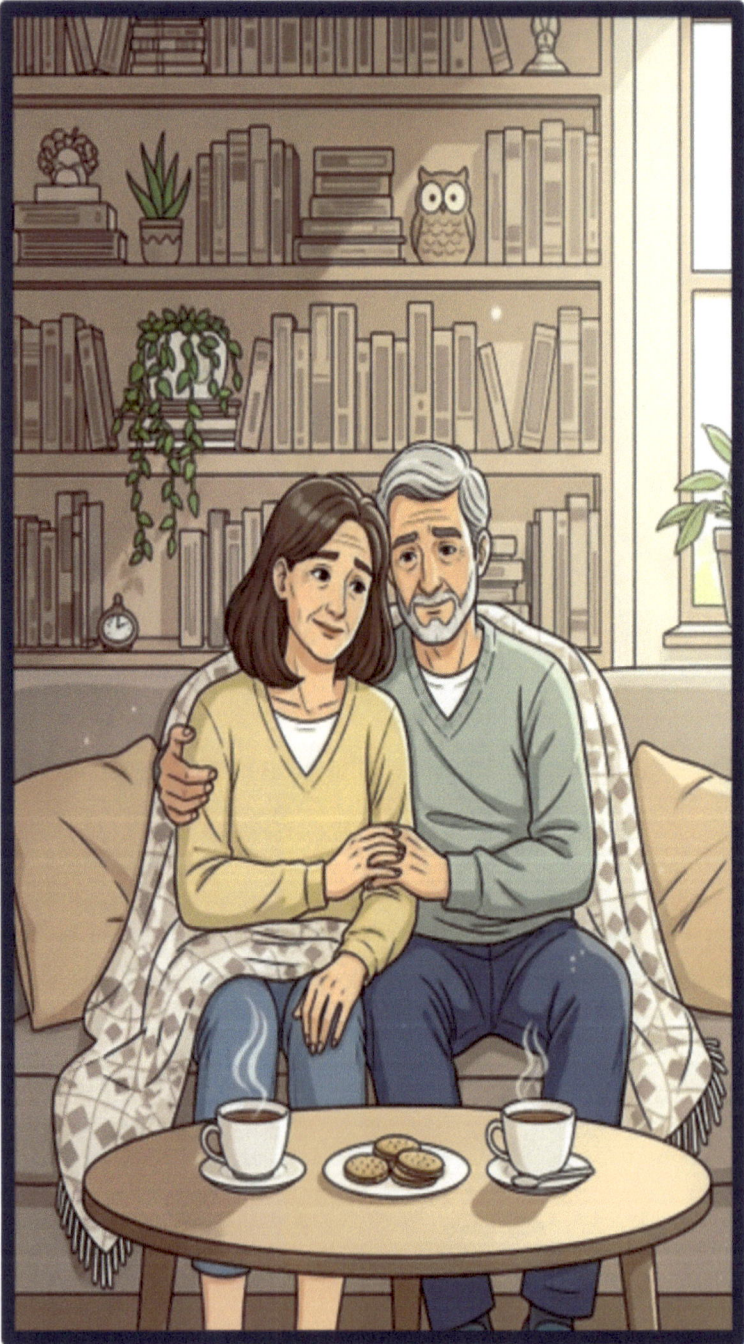

Chapter 4: Supporting Each Other Through This Challenge

Supporting your partner through ED while taking care of yourself isn't just possible-it's essential!

I learned this the hard way during my struggle, watching her try to find the balance between being supportive and losing herself in my health challenges.

Let me share what I discovered about what real support looks like, why taking care of yourself helps your partner, and how to build the foundation that will serve your relationship long after ED is resolved.

What I Actually Needed From Her

When my ED started, she immediately went into what I now call "super-support mode." She became my cheerleader, researcher, and emotional manager all rolled into one. Her heart was completely in the right place, but what I needed was simpler and more sustainable.

Being My Stable Presence

During those months when everything felt uncertain about my body and our intimate future, she became my constant. This didn't mean she suppressed her own emotions, but she didn't make my worst moments about her needs in that moment.

I remember one particularly rough evening after my pills failed again. I was spiraling into shame and self-criticism, convinced I was broken beyond repair. Instead of trying to talk me out of my emotions or fix my mood, she simply sat with me and told me this was hard, and she was there.

That presence meant everything. She stayed steady when I had setbacks, didn't try to talk me out of difficult emotions immediately, maintained consistent affection regardless of how my body was performing, and avoided dramatic reactions to treatment news.

The Pressure I Didn't Realize She Was Creating

There's a fine line between supportive encouragement and pressure that creates additional stress. She meant well, but I started noticing that some of her encouragement made me worse.

When she'd get excited about new treatments or tell me how proud she was of trying new approaches, it tied her pride and optimism to my medical success. That meant if treatment failed, I wasn't just disappointing my body, I was disappointing her expectations.

What helped more was when she celebrated who I was rather than what I was accomplishing. When she told me she was proud of how I was handling this challenge or that she believed in us whatever happened, it removed the burden of having to succeed to earn her continued support.

Maintaining Our Normal Life

One of the most supportive things she did was refuse to let ED consume our entire relationship. She insisted we continue activities, conversations, and traditions that had nothing to do with sexual performance or this situation.

When she maintained this normalcy, she reminded me that I was still the same person she fell in love with, health struggles and all. We weren't just partners facing ED. We were a couple who happened to be navigating this while living a full life together.

Learning Our Limits Together

But even with all this support, something wasn't working. For the first few months, she tried to carry everything. She researched treatments, managed my emotions, and basically made my struggle her full-time job. I could see the exhaustion building in her eyes, but I didn't know how to tell her to stop helping without sounding ungrateful.

The breaking point came one evening when she handed me a stack of printouts about a new supplement she'd found. She told me she'd spent three hours researching it that day, hoping maybe this one would work better than the pills.

I looked at her tired face and realized something had to change. We needed to figure out what was her responsibility and what was mine.

Finding What Worked for Both of Us

I discovered she felt guilty about not wanting to research every possible treatment, and I felt guilty about needing help but also needing space. We started being honest about what she could realistically handle without losing herself.

She laid it out clearly. She could be there for me emotionally, but she couldn't make my health challenge her personal project. She loved me, but she wasn't qualified to be my doctor, researcher, and therapist all at once.

Through trial and error, we found our balance. When I needed to discuss my fears or frustrations, she listened. Doctor's appointments were something she could attend when I asked, but I needed to handle scheduling them and asking the questions. She could celebrate small victories with me and comfort me during setbacks.

But there were things she realized she couldn't do sustainability. She couldn't absorb my emotions as if they were her own. When I was having a terrible day, she could comfort me, but she didn't have to experience terrible emotions too. She couldn't research every treatment option and present me with solutions. That became my responsibility.

She also couldn't put her entire life on hold while we worked through this. She needed to keep seeing friends, pursuing her interests, and taking care of her own health. She put it perfectly when she told me she was my girlfriend, not my medical case manager.

Why Her Self-Care Actually Helped Me

The most surprising thing I discovered: when she took care of herself, it helped me heal. When she neglected her own well-being to focus entirely on supporting me, it made everything worse for both of us.

When she prioritized her own well-being, exercising regularly, maintaining friendships, pursuing interests, she demonstrated that focusing on health wasn't selfish. This gave me permission to prioritize my own healing without guilt.

She protected her basics: adequate sleep, physical activity, and nutrition. She protected her joy: continuing activities that brought happiness, staying connected with supportive people, and pursuing creative outlets.

When physical intimacy in our relationship became complicated, she even got professional massages to meet her need for healthy, non-sexual touch. At first, I wondered about this, but then I realized it was brilliant, she was taking care of her needs without putting pressure on me.

Later she told me that when she started taking better care of herself, it reminded both of us that this challenge didn't have to consume our entire lives.

She Came Back from Choice, Not Obligation

For several months early on, she had sacrificed everything to focus on supporting me. She gave up activities she enjoyed, declined social invitations, and made my struggle the center of her entire existence. Within a few months, I could sense her resentment building, even though she tried to hide it.

When she started reclaiming her own interests and social life, any resentment disappeared. She came back to our relationship from choice rather than martyrdom, which was so much better for both of us.

Her boundaries weren't walls to keep me out-they were guidelines that helped us both know how to show up for each other without either of us losing ourselves in the process.

What We Built Together

Successfully navigating ED as a team created something precious: absolute knowledge that our love could withstand genuine difficulty. We weren't just surviving a health challenge. We were strengthening a bond that would serve us for a lifetime.

We discovered forms of intimacy that didn't depend on sexual function. We proved we could handle anything life brought as a team. Before ED, we'd operated on relationship autopilot. ED woke us up to how precious and fragile our connection really was.

Now we're much more intentional about nurturing our relationship. We schedule regular connection time, express appreciation explicitly, and check in regularly about relationship satisfaction.

She didn't become cold or unsupportive when she established guidelines. She became thoughtfully supportive. Instead of trying to fix everything, she focused on loving me through the uncertainty. Instead of trying to solve my problem, she helped create a safe space where we could both be honest about what we were experiencing.

What This Might Look Like for You

Your boundaries might be different from ours, but the principle is the same: you can be incredibly supportive without making his situation your personal project. You can love him deeply while still protecting your own well-being.

The key is being honest about what you can give sustainably, not what you think you should be able to handle. Taking care of yourself isn't selfish. This is what allows you to show up as a genuine partner rather than a burned-out caregiver.

The experience you're sharing while facing ED isn't just recovery from a medical challenge. It's conscious creation of the relationship you want for your lifetime together. You're growing into something more beautiful and intentional than what you had before.

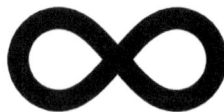

∞

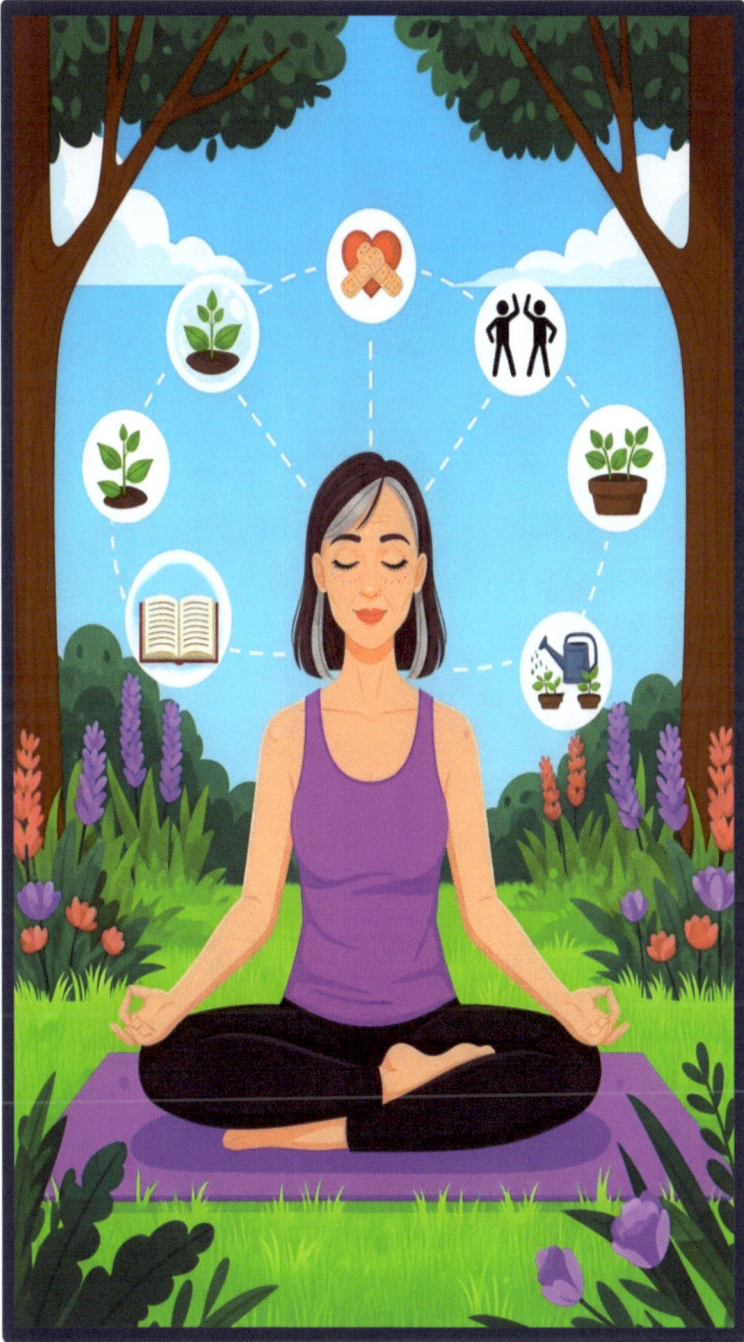

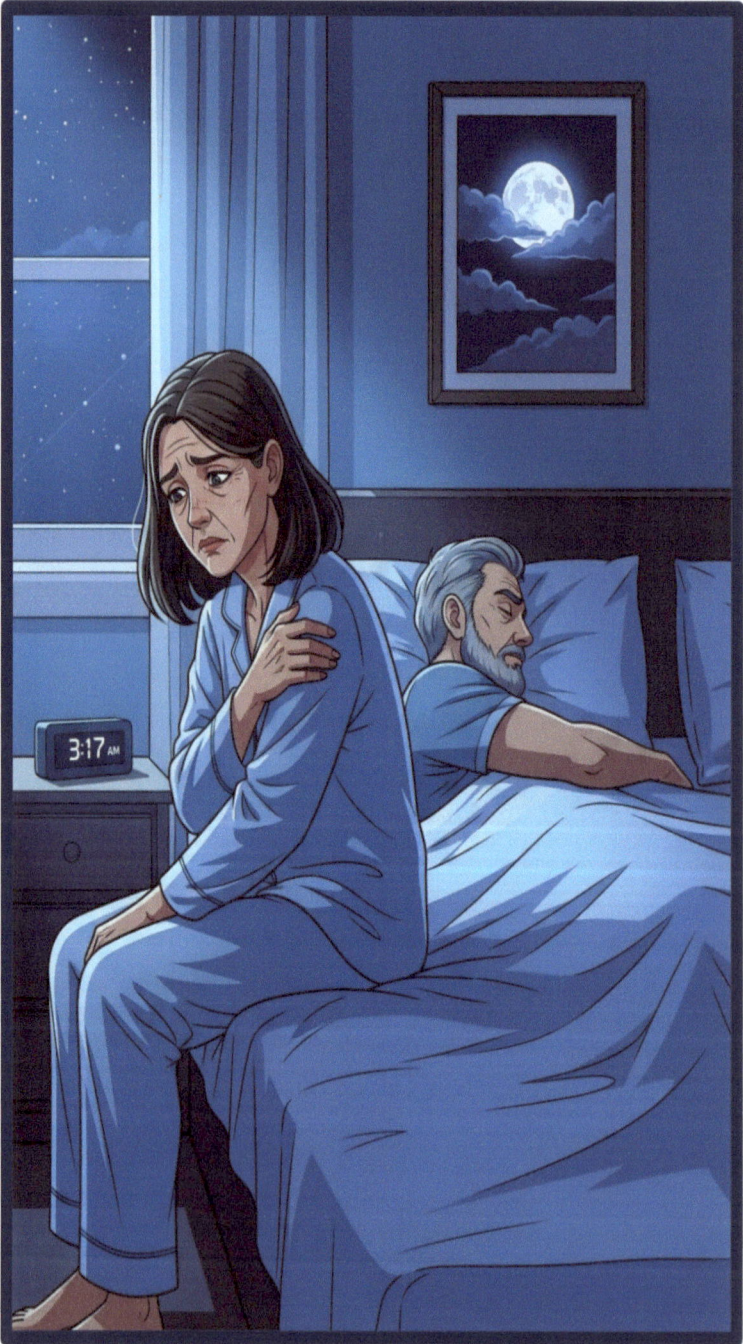

Chapter 5: The Questions That Keep You Awake

Let me tackle some thoughts that may be keeping you up at night, the ones that feel too awkward to voice out loud, the worries that make you question everything about yourself and your relationship. I've been there, and more importantly, I've watched my partner wrestle with these exact same fears.

These aren't just normal concerns; they're the essential questions that every woman facing ED needs answered.

When Your Body Still Wants What His Can't Give

My partner tortured herself over this for months. She wanted sexual connection while I was struggling, and that made her feel selfish and insensitive. But she believed she could turn off her sexuality, like turning off a light, because my plumbing was broken, and she did.

Most men with ED still want intimacy. We still want to connect with you, still want to please you, even when our bodies won't cooperate the way we want them to. The key became having those awkward but necessary conversations about what felt good for both of us.

You're wanting him isn't weird or insensitive. It's normal and healthy.

The Sexual Frustration No One Talks About

This might be the most important issue she never felt comfortable discussing. She was silent about this for months, thinking she had to sacrifice her needs to support mine. That's not sustainable, and it's not fair to either of you.

The breakthrough came when she realized that taking care of her needs wasn't selfish. It was essential for supporting me effectively. When she was sexually frustrated and resentful, it created tension neither of us needed.

Working together, we discovered new ways of being close that satisfied both of us without putting pressure on my performance. She also found healthy outlets for her sexual energy through massages that didn't involve me at all. At first, I wondered about this, but then I realized it took pressure off me while helping her stay balanced.

The frustration you're experiencing is real and valid. Don't let it build into resentment by suffering in silence.

The Fear That Things Will Never Be Normal Again

She'd stay up at night wondering if our intimate life would ever feel natural again. She'd think about how spontaneous and easy things used to be, then look at our current reality of planning, timing medications, and managing expectations.

Your intimate life probably won't be exactly the same, but here's the surprising part: it might end up better. Our sexual relationship now is more intentional, more communicative, and way more creative than it ever was before ED.

We learned to express what we wanted instead of just assuming. We became more present with each other instead of going through the motions. We began to define intimacy in broader ways than just intercourse.

ED forced us to discover forms of connection we'd never explored before. Even after my function came back, we kept many of the practices we'd learned because they made our intimacy richer. Sometimes what feels like the worst thing that could happen to your sex life ends up teaching you things you never would have learned otherwise.

Watching Him Disappear Emotionally

As we discussed in Chapter 2, ED hits men right in their sense of identity and self-worth, so depression becomes a real risk. She learned to watch for warning signs that went beyond just sexual withdrawal: when I started pulling back from everything, not just sex, when I lost interest in things I used to enjoy, when I couldn't shake emotions of hopelessness or worthlessness.

The most important thing she did was normalize my difficult emotions while staying alert for signs that I needed more help than she could provide. She didn't try to talk me out of bad days, but she also didn't let me disappear entirely.

If you're worried about depression taking over, encourage him to talk to someone who specializes in helping people through these challenges. Sometimes you need professional help to sort through the emotional mess that ED can create. Your love and support matter enormously, but they can't replace professional guidance when depression gets involved.

The Timeline Question Everyone's Afraid to Ask

Sometimes she would do mental math: *"It's been three months... six months... how long is too long?"* She'd research online, looking for some magical number that would tell her when to worry or when to feel hopeful.

Here's the truth nobody wants to hear: there's no magic timeline. Some guys get lucky, and the first treatment works within a few weeks. Others spend months trying different approaches before something clicks. I wish I could give you a specific number, but ED doesn't follow a schedule.

Measuring success by asking *"Is he fixed yet?"* will drive you both crazy. She had to shift her thinking completely. Instead of waiting for me to be *"cured,"* she started celebrating the smaller wins: when I seemed more hopeful, when we talked more openly, when I stopped avoiding physical affection altogether.

Your role isn't to promise quick results or keep track of how long this is taking. Your role is to be the steady presence while he rides the ups and downs of whatever treatment he is trying. Some days will feel like progress; others will feel like setbacks. That's normal, even when treatment is working.

The hardest part for her was learning that *"getting better"* doesn't happen in a straight line. There were good days that gave us hope, followed by terrible days that made us feel like we were back at square one. But looking back now, I can see that even during the setbacks, we were building something stronger together.

The Secret Worry About Your Own Needs

There's another question I know you're thinking but might not voice: *"Am I terrible for struggling with this too?"* The answer is absolutely not. Remember: ED doesn't just happen to him; it happens to both of you.

Your confusion, sadness, frustration, even anger-those are natural responses to watching your intimate life get turned upside down. She went through her own grief process. She mourned the spontaneous intimacy we'd lost, worried about our future, questioned whether she was still desirable to me. All of those emotions were completely valid and normal.

Self-care isn't selfish when you're supporting someone through a health challenge. It's what equips you to show up with genuine love instead of depleted obligation. Taking time for your friendships, your health, your hobbies-that's not abandoning him. That's making sure you have something left to give.

Moving Forward Together

Every worry you've been afraid to voice is valid. The fact that you're here, looking for answers, shows how much you care. You don't need to be perfect at this. You just need to be present, patient, and willing to figure it out together.

You're not alone in this experience, and your emotions matter just as much as his do. The questions that feel selfish or awkward? Those are often the most important ones to address. Don't suffer in silence when you could be building something stronger together.

Your concerns about sex, frustration, timelines, his mental health, and your own needs, they are all part of navigating this challenge as a team. The couples who come out stronger aren't the ones who never have these worries; they're the ones who face them honestly and work through them together.

"Intimacy isn't lost when bodies falter;

it's lost when hearts stop reaching for each other."

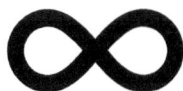

∞

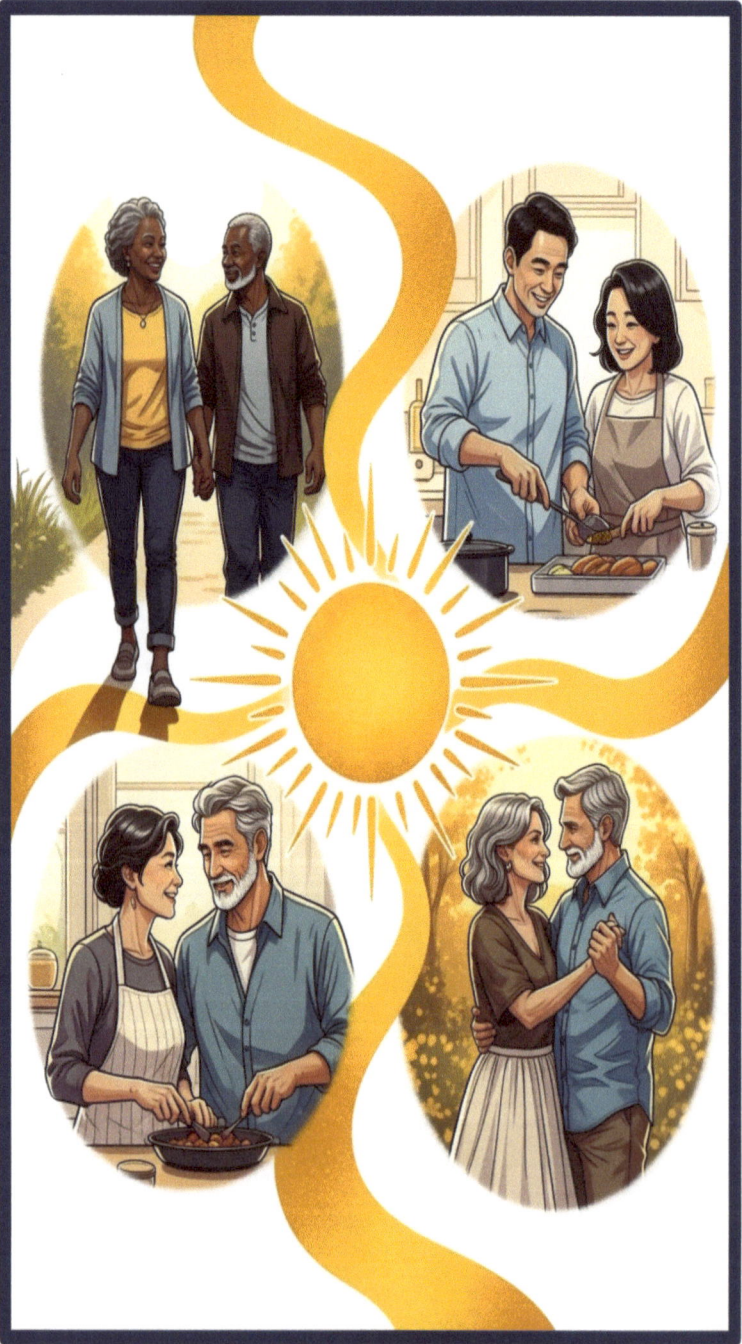

Chapter 6: Success Stories and Building Your Future

When you're in the thick of this challenge, it can feel like life will never be normal again. I remember those dark months when the silence, the frustration, and the distance between my partner and me felt permanent. But what I've discovered since then, through my own experience and through conversations with other couples, is that this struggle often becomes a turning point that transforms relationships in ways no one expects.

Let me share some stories from other couples who've reached out to me. They might not mirror yours exactly, but their paths toward hope and healing offer lessons that could guide your own experience.

Sarah and Mike: Building Early Strength

Sarah (28) and Mike (30) met ED early in their two-year relationship. Mike's problems began when work stress escalated, then worsened after he started taking antidepressants for anxiety.

When I first talked with Sarah, she was desperate. She felt like they were too young for this, thinking ED only happened to older people with relationship problems. She couldn't understand how this could be happening to them.

Mike's shame was consuming him. He felt like he was failing as a man and as a boyfriend, so he started avoiding intimacy entirely because he couldn't handle disappointing her again.

What saved their relationship was seeking help early before the silence and distance had time to solidify. A therapist helped them understand that ED affects men of any age and that their responses, Sarah's confusion and self-blame, Mike's withdrawal and shame, were completely normal.

More importantly, they separated sexual performance from intimate connection. They discovered ways to maintain closeness and pleasure that didn't depend on erections working perfectly every time.

Mike eventually found success with ED pills.

When I spoke with them a few months later, what impressed me most was how the communication skills they'd developed served them through other challenges: job changes, family stress, financial concerns.

Sarah later told me that going through ED together taught them they could handle anything. They learned to discuss difficult topics before they became crises.

Their breakthrough: Early intervention, both medical and emotional, creates an ability to bounce back that extends far beyond sexual health. When couples address it promptly and honestly, they often build stronger partnerships than they had before.

Lisa and David: Finding Each Other Again

David's story reminded me of my own experience. After 15 years of marriage, his blood pressure medication triggered ED. What started as an assumed temporary side effect stretched into months of confusion and growing distance.

Lisa began questioning everything: her attractiveness, their connection, whether he still wanted her. Meanwhile, David was watching her self-doubt grow while feeling powerless to reassure her physically. The guilt was eating him alive.

Their breakthrough came through a conversation that could have destroyed them but instead saved their marriage. Lisa finally said it directly: that she felt like he didn't want her anymore.

David's response shocked her as she had no idea what was happening. He wanted her more than ever, but he was embarrassed that his body wasn't working. He didn't know how to show her that this wasn't about her.

That moment of raw honesty opened the door to real communication. They started approaching treatment as a team instead of him struggling alone while she wondered what she'd done wrong.

When pills continued to provide inconsistent results, David chose implant surgery. A decision they made together after months of research and discussion. The recovery period became an unexpected gift, giving them uninterrupted time for deeper conversations about aging, dreams, and appreciation for their life together.

A year later, both report their intimate life surpasses what they had before ED emerged. They discuss everything now. Not just sex, but their fears, their needs, their hopes for the future. ED forced them to become real partners instead of just people who happened to be married.

What they discovered: Honest communication transforms relationship difficulties into opportunities for deeper connection. Thriving couples don't avoid difficult conversations; they learn to have them with love and respect.

Jennifer and Robert: When Everything Goes Wrong at Once

Sometimes ED gets complicated by other issues, and Jennifer and Robert's tale proves that even complex situations can have hopeful outcomes. Robert's ED coincided with Jennifer discovering his pornography use, creating a perfect storm of medical and trust issues.

Jennifer couldn't understand how he could have problems with her but not with porn. She felt rejected and betrayed, like proof that she wasn't enough for him.

Robert was drowning in shame about both issues. He was embarrassed about the ED and guilty about the porn. He felt like he was failing Jennifer in every possible way. The pornography had become his way of dealing with sexual anxiety, but it was making everything worse.

Through intensive therapy, they addressed both issues simultaneously rebuilding emotional intimacy while pursuing medical treatment for ED. It was messy, painful work that took nearly two years.

When I spoke with them recently, they described having the most honest, intimate relationship either had ever experienced. Robert told me that working through these problems together taught them they could handle anything. They realized that difficulties don't have to destroy relationships, they can actually strengthen them if you face them together.

Their hard-won wisdom: Even when ED is complicated by other relationship issues, couples can successfully rebuild both trust and intimacy. Professional guidance and unwavering commitment to honesty make the difference between relationships that fracture and relationships that heal.

What I've Seen Across All These Stories

Talking with these couples and other friends who have navigated ED successfully, I see certain patterns that offer hope for anyone currently struggling:

- **Treatment really does work.** With current medical options, most men can regain sexual function. Sometimes it takes trying multiple approaches, and the timeline varies dramatically, but persistence pays off. Incidentally, I know treatment works. I went the full gamut, pills/herbs, injections, vacuum pump, and finally the implant which works 100% of the time.

- **Communication transforms everything.** Every successful couple I've spoken with developed skills for discussing their fears, needs, and hopes openly. This ability doesn't just help with ED; it revolutionizes every aspect of their relationship.

- **Redefining intimacy opens new doors.** When couples explore connection beyond intercourse, many discover forms of intimacy they never would have tried otherwise. Emotional vulnerability and creative physical connection can thrive even when sex changes.

- **The struggle becomes the teacher.** I've yet to meet someone who would choose to go through ED, but many tell me they're grateful for what it taught them about love, resilience, and partnership.

The Truth About Thriving Together

The relationships that thrive don't do so because they avoid hardship. They thrive because they face difficulty together with honesty, patience, and determination to emerge stronger. They discuss the impossible topics. They care for themselves and each other. They respect each others healing process. They choose to nurture love even when intimacy becomes complicated.

During my darkest months with ED, I couldn't imagine that our relationship would not only survive but become deeper and more resilient than before. Yet that's exactly what happened, and I've witnessed the same transformation with many other couples.

ED doesn't have to be the end of your closeness. In fact, for many couples, it becomes the doorway to a deeper, more conscious, more intentionally connected relationship than they ever thought possible.

What you've created while facing ED together, the deeper understanding, genuine intimacy, and unshakable trust you've developed, will carry you through anything life brings your way.

"Love grows strongest not when things are easy, but when two people choose to keep walking forward through the hard."

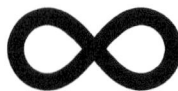

∞

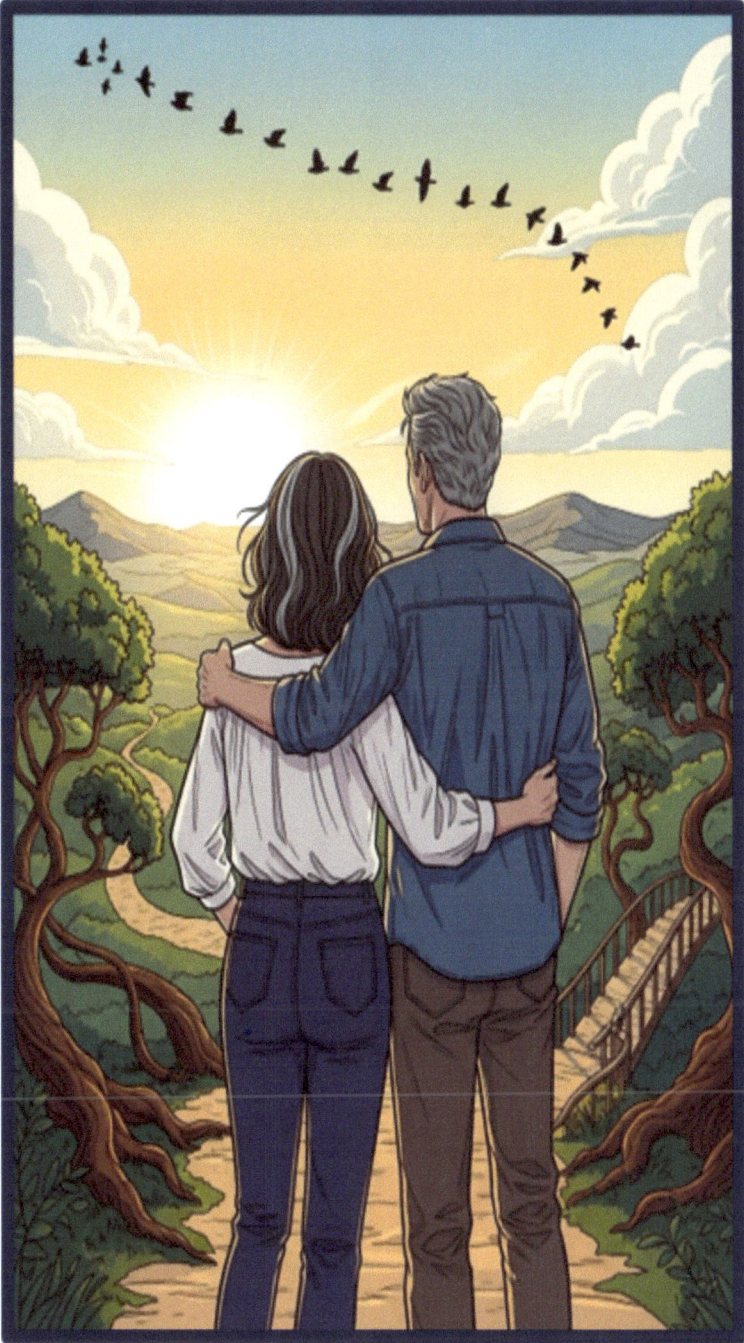

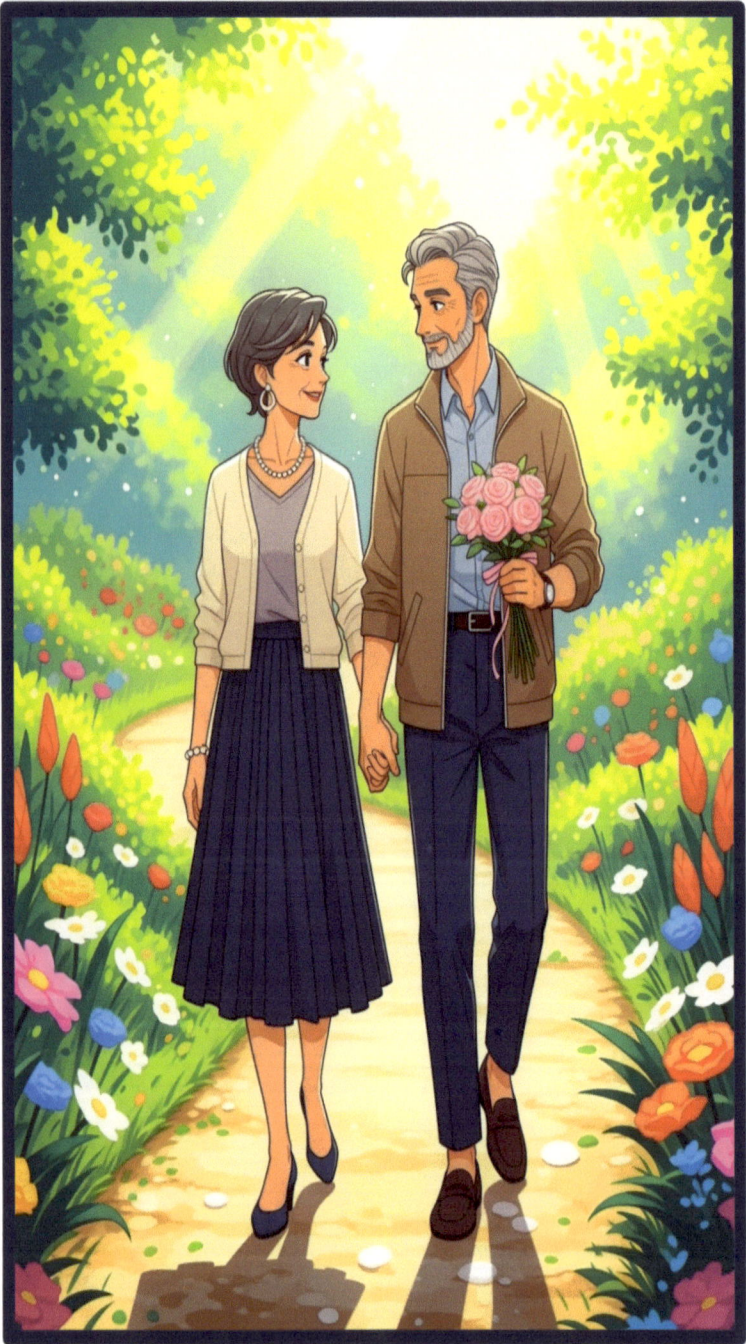

Chapter 7: When Treatment Works

The phone rang Thursday afternoon after my surgery. "The surgery went perfectly," my doctor said. "You should be back to full function in about six to eight weeks."

After years of struggling with ED, I finally had a penile implant. This was the solution I'd been working toward. I should have felt pure relief, but instead, I found myself sitting in my bedroom with tears in my eyes, overwhelmed by emotions I hadn't expected.

I've shared the complete story of my personal ED experience, from the first failed pills through trying every possible treatment before choosing surgery, in my first book: *"When Pills Stop Working, A Complete Guide to Advanced Solutions for Men"*. That book walks through the medical side of what I went through. This one focuses on what both of us experienced together.

If you're reading this chapter, you and your partner may be approaching or experiencing treatment success. Whether it's pills that finally work consistently, injections that restore function, or surgery like mine, both of you have earned this moment.

But if you're finding that "success" feels more complicated than you imagined, you're not alone. Recovery brings its own surprises that no one discusses.

The Surprise of Success

When I came home from implant surgery, my partner's reaction caught me off guard. Instead of pure celebration, I saw relief mixed with something that looked almost like worry. She told me she was happy but also scared to hope too much. What if something went wrong? What if this didn't work the way we thought it would?

After so many disappointments with other treatments, both of us had built emotional armor by not expecting too much. We'd gotten good at being cautiously hopeful, at bracing for setbacks, at not counting on anything working perfectly. That protection didn't just fall away because the medical solution was finally in place.

During my recovery period, she told me something that made perfect sense: "I keep waiting for the other shoe to drop. I've gotten so used to tiptoeing around ED that suddenly not having to feels strange." Both of us had developed habits, being extra careful around intimacy, managing our hopes like fragile things-that took time to let go of even after successful treatment.

You've probably been through so much disappointment that trusting good news feels scary. That protective caution isn't negativity; it's wisdom both of you have earned during this difficult experience.

When Your Body Remembers What Your Mind Forgot

Even after my implant was working perfectly, I sometimes felt what I started calling "ghost anxiety." My device worked flawlessly, but my mind would occasionally spiral into familiar fears during intimate moments. All those months of performance anxiety had worn deep paths in my brain that took time to heal.

She noticed her own version of this. Despite my body working consistently, she sometimes caught herself watching my face during intimacy, looking for signs that something might go wrong. The watchfulness both of us had developed during our struggle didn't disappear overnight just because treatment worked.

"I had to teach my brain to trust what was happening," she told me months later. "Even when everything was working wonderfully, part of me was still holding my breath." This isn't a sign that something's wrong with your recovery, it's proof of how deeply this experience affected both your hearts.

Rediscovering Spontaneity

For so long, we'd approached intimacy like following a medical protocol. We timed everything around medications, managed our expectations carefully, and planned for different outcomes. When my implant made spontaneous intimacy possible again, we realized we'd almost forgotten how to just let things happen naturally.

I'll never forget our first truly unplanned intimate moment after months of careful orchestration. It felt strange to just follow our desires without checking our mental lists of what might go wrong. Both of us had to consciously remember how to trust our bodies and our bond.

She had her own adjustment to make. *"I had to remember that I could reach for you,"* she shared. *"I'd become so careful about not creating pressure that I'd almost stopped showing my own desires."*

The wonderful part about finding spontaneity again is that it builds on itself. It started small, a kiss that lasted longer than usual, touching just because it felt good, letting affection grow without planning where it would lead.

Her Emotional Journey Continues

While I was celebrating my restored body, she was still carrying months of hurt, confusion, and exhaustion. My surgical success didn't magically erase the emotional bruises she'd collected during our worst times.

"I needed time to believe this was real," she told me months later. *"And I needed to deal with all the feelings I'd buried while I was trying to be strong for you."* Her heart needed its own timeline for healing, and I had to honor that.

During the crisis, we'd poured everything into just surviving, there wasn't room to fully feel the weight of months of rejection, the loss of easy intimacy, or the exhaustion of constantly worrying. When treatment worked and the immediate crisis passed, all those emotions finally surfaced.

We needed honest conversations about the hurt and fear that had been pushed aside. Don't skip this part: mending your heart is just as important as fixing the physical problem.

We also discovered what I call *"success pressure"*, thinking that since treatment has worked, everything should be perfect immediately. We'd get frustrated when normal relationship stuff came up or when intimacy wasn't magical every single time. *"We fixed this,"* we'd think, *"so why isn't everything amazing now?"*

Recovery means weaving successful treatment into regular life, which still includes ordinary ups and downs and the reality that no relationship is perfect all the time, even with perfect sexual function.

Rebuilding Confidence Together

My implant worked perfectly from day one, but that didn't automatically restore our confidence as lovers. I had to trust my new body, and she had to trust our intimate bond again after so many months of disappointment.

We celebrated the small victories:

- The first time we were together, without me obsessing over whether everything was working.

- The first time she initiated, without that flash of worry in her eyes.

- The first time we laughed during sex instead of holding our breath and hoping.

Rebuilding confidence meant discussing the healing process, not just the medical results. I'd share when I felt those phantom worries creeping in. She'd tell me when she noticed herself bracing for problems that couldn't happen anymore. We celebrated together when intimacy felt easy and natural again.

Creating Your New Normal

The connection we developed after my implant wasn't the same one, we had before ED. Both of us had changed and grown during those tough months. Our intimate life now included everything we had discovered about communicating openly, being emotionally close, and supporting each other through uncertainty.

We gained new ways to share our desires and concerns. We discovered forms of closeness that went beyond just sexual performance.

Your new normal will be uniquely yours, but it'll likely be more thoughtful and intentional than what you had before. That awareness is something precious that grew from your struggle together.

What caught me off guard most about our new normal was how it changed what we considered "successful" intimacy. This shift didn't happen overnight-it evolved as we realized that our old way of measuring intimate success felt too narrow for the deeper relationship we'd become.

Expanding Your Definition of Success

Before ED, our intimate life followed a familiar pattern: attraction led to foreplay, foreplay led to intercourse, intercourse led to climax, and that meant success. When my implant made reliable intercourse possible again, we discovered we'd developed much richer ways to measure intimate success.

One thing that surprised us after successful treatment was feeling almost guilty about enjoying other forms of intimacy. I remember the first time we chose extended touching and mutual pleasure without intercourse, even though my implant meant intercourse was easily available. For a moment, I wondered, *"Should we be having 'real' sex since we can now?"*

She felt something similar. *"I felt strange sometimes preferring other kinds of intimacy,"* she told me. *"Like I was wasting the opportunity we'd fought so hard to get back."*

We had to consciously give ourselves permission to enjoy the full range of intimate experiences we'd discovered, not just intercourse.

We'd realized that closeness, pleasure, communication, and mutual satisfaction mattered more than any specific physical performance. Even with perfect function restored, we sometimes chose forms of intimacy we'd discovered during our ED experience, not because we had to, but because we genuinely loved the variety and emotional depth, they brought us.

"I realized I'd been measuring our intimacy by your erection instead of by how close we felt," she told me. *"Now I measure it by our bond, laughter, satisfaction, and how loved I feel afterward."*

Expanding your definition of success doesn't mean settling for less-it means recognizing that intimate satisfaction has many expressions and embracing that variety makes your relationship more resilient and satisfying.

Your Intimate Future

Navigating ED together has created something deeper and more genuine than you imagined.

You've proven that love adapts, grows, and deepens through difficulty. You've discovered that true intimacy includes emotional vulnerability, mutual pleasure, creative exploration, and genuine partnership. You've found that your bond is strong enough to weather serious challenges and emerge more intimate than before.

Most importantly, you've created something that can handle whatever future challenges arise. The skills you developed will serve you through anything life brings.

Your intimate future is brighter than you can see right now. The love that carried you through ED is strong enough to carry you through anything.

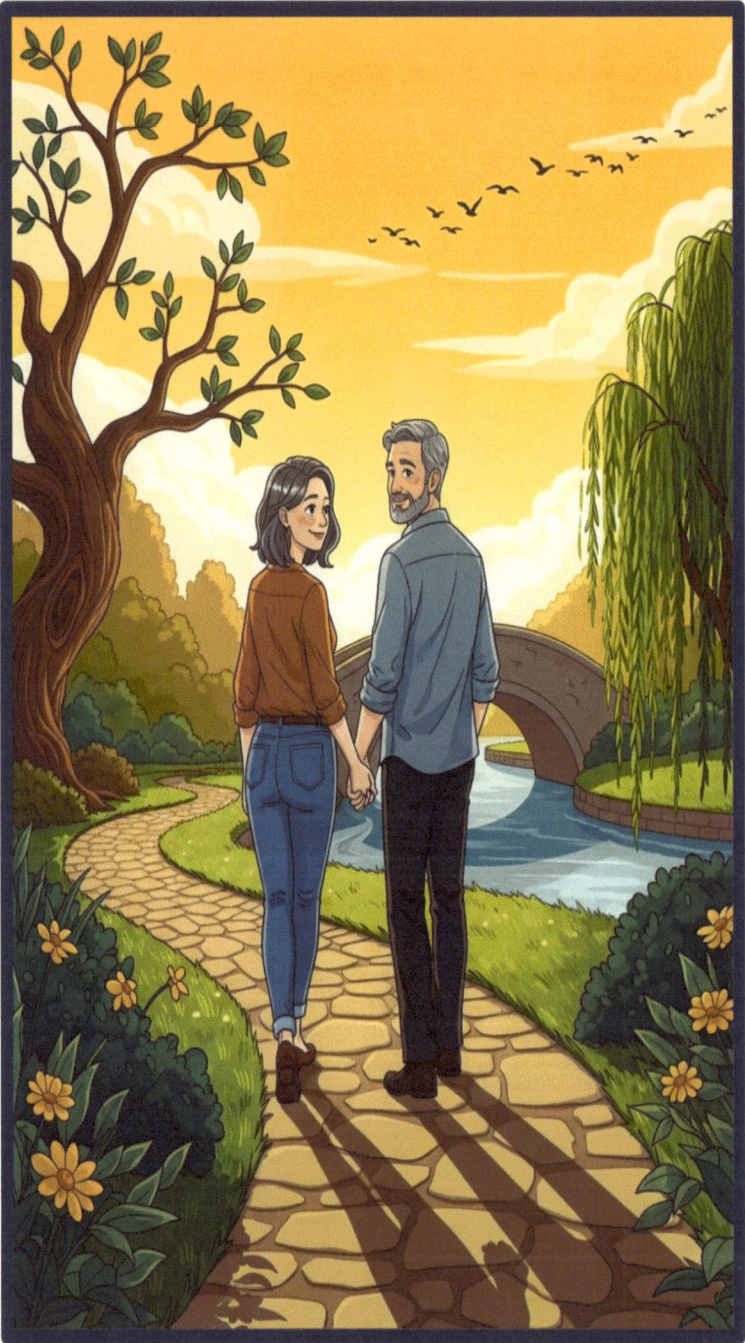

Conclusion: Your Story Continues

I'm sitting here thinking about you as I write this final chapter. I picture you reading this late at night when the house is quiet, or stealing a few minutes during your lunch break, or curled up on your couch on a Sunday afternoon. Wherever you are, I hope you feel a little less alone than when you started this book.

When I was going through what you're experiencing now, I wished desperately that someone would just tell my partner the truth: that what she was experiencing was normal, that it wasn't her fault, and that we were going to be okay. I couldn't give her that certainty then because I didn't have it myself. But I can give it to you now.

You're Going to Be Okay

Not just *survive okay*, maybe even better than okay.

I know that sounds impossible right now, especially if you're in those dark weeks where everything seems broken and you can't see past the next failed attempt at intimacy. But what I've learned from my own experience and from conversations with other couples is this: this chapter of your story has an ending, and it's a good one.

The woman reading this book right now, the one who's scared and confused but still searching for answers, she's the same woman who's going to look back on this time and be proud of how she handled it. You're going to see that your strength carried both of you through something really hard.

What I Want You to Remember

- **You didn't cause this.** I know you know that intellectually, but I need you to feel it in your bones. Nothing you did, didn't do, said, or didn't say created this situation. ED happens to good men in happy relationships all the time.

- **Your emotions matter just as much as his.** You don't have to be the endlessly patient, understanding partner who never has bad days. You're allowed to be frustrated, sad, confused, or even angry sometimes. That doesn't make you unsupportive: it makes you human.

- **You're not alone in these experiences.** Right now, thousands of other women are wondering if their relationship will survive this, questioning their attractiveness, researching treatments at 2 AM, and struggling with guilt for having sexual needs while their partner struggles.

- **You are part of a club nobody wants to join**, but the membership comes with the knowledge that others have walked this path and made it through.

The Secret I Learned

Something I couldn't have understood during our worst months: ED didn't ruin our relationship. It revealed what our relationship was really made of. And what we discovered under all that pressure and fear was something amazing.

We learned we could discuss anything. We figured out how to support each other through genuine difficulty. We discovered that love isn't just the easy moments, it's choosing each other when things get complicated.

The relationship we have now is more solid than what we had before, not because we went through something terrible, but because we went through it together without giving up on each other.

Your Relationship is Stronger Than You Think

I bet if someone asked you right now to list your relationship's strengths, you'd struggle to come up with much. When ED moves in, it has a way of making everything else fade into the background. But think about what brought you two together in the first place. Think about the laughs you've shared, the way he looks at you when you're not paying attention, the inside jokes, the way you work as a team on regular problems.

All of that is still there. ED is loud and demanding and makes you forget, but your foundation hasn't disappeared. You're just building on it now in ways you never expected.

What's Coming

- Treatment will work. Maybe not the first thing you try, maybe not as quickly as you want, but it will happen. The medical options available now are remarkable, and most men find something that helps if they keep trying.

- But even before that happens, things are going to start getting lighter. The conversations will become easier. You'll have more good days than bad ones. You'll start sleeping better. You'll remember what it's like to just enjoy being together without that constant worry humming in the background.

- And when treatment does work, when you're on the other side of this, you're going to have something precious: absolute proof that your love can handle anything life throws at you.

A Note from My Heart to Yours

If we were sitting together over coffee right now, this is what I'd want you to know: You're handling this better than you think you are. The fact that you picked up this book, that you're fighting for your relationship, that you're trying to understand and support while also taking care of yourself, that takes real courage.

Your partner is lucky to have you. Not because you're perfect or because you never struggle, but because you're choosing to stay and figure this out together.

This season of your life is hard, but it's not your whole story. Your best chapters, the ones where you look at each other and smile about how far you've come, where intimacy is natural and joyful again, where you barely remember what it was like to be this worried, those chapters are coming.

Until then, be gentle with yourself. Trust the process. Keep communicating with each other. And remember that every day you don't give up is a day closer to the breakthrough that's waiting for you.

You've got this. And more importantly, you've got each other.

That's enough.

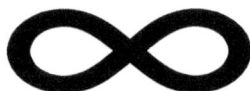

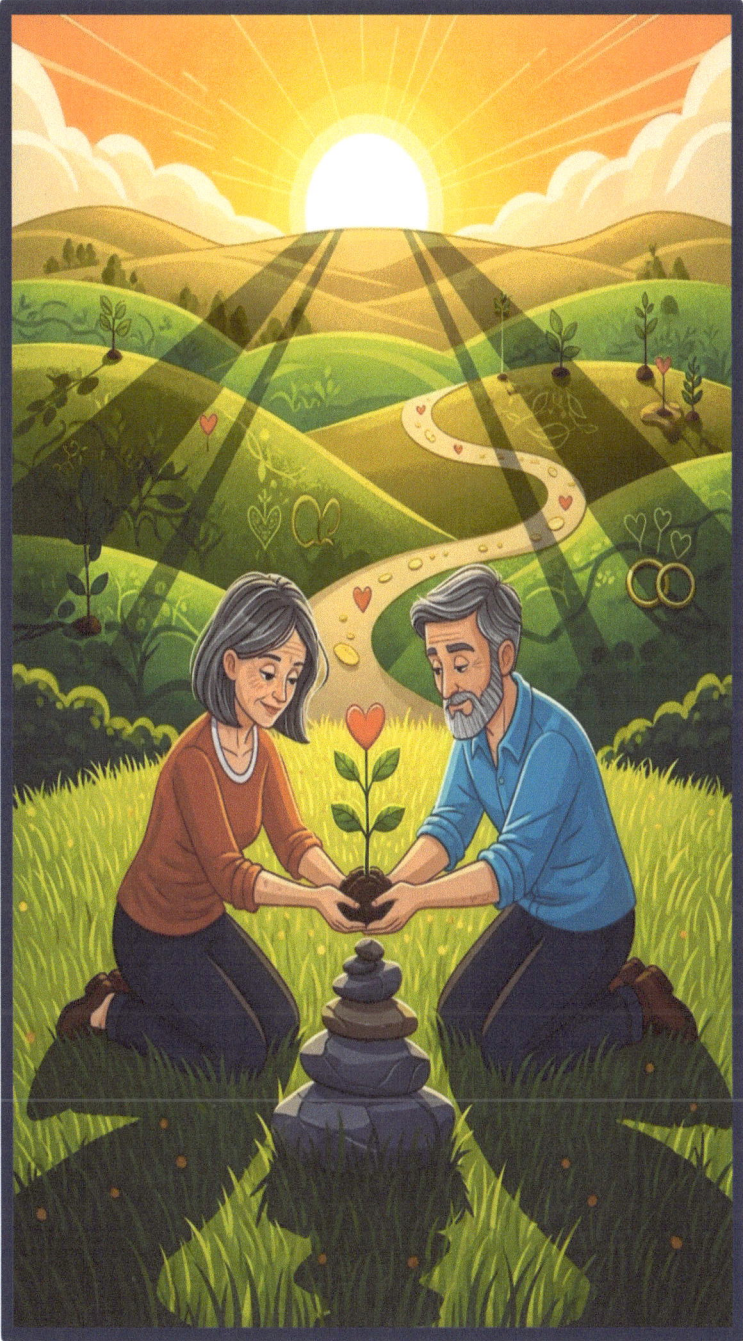

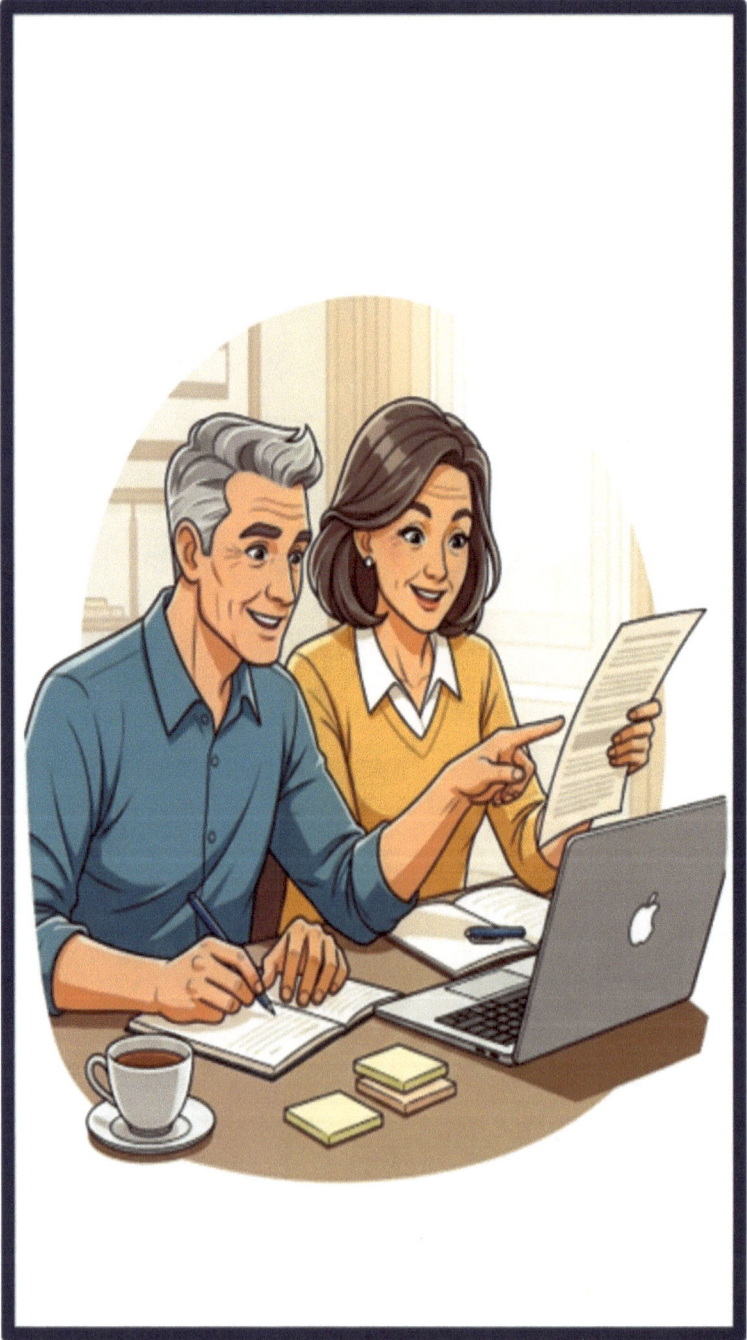

Resources

When my partner and I were first navigating ED, we felt overwhelmed by the amount of information available online. Some sources were helpful, others made us more confused, and many weren't written with partners in mind. I've compiled this list of resources that we found genuinely useful, along with some I wish we'd discovered sooner.

Remember, you don't need to research everything at once. Start with what feels most relevant to your situation right now.

Medical Information and Treatment

Understanding the medical side of ED helped both of us stop feeling so helpless. These resources provide reliable, current information without the fear-mongering you'll find on some websites.

Primary Medical Organizations:

- National Institute of Diabetes and Digestive and Kidney Diseases (NIDDK):

    www.niddk.nih.gov

- American Urological Association:

    www.auanet.org

- Sexual Medicine Society of North America:

    www.smsna.org

- Cleveland Clinic Erectile Dysfunction Information:
    my.clevelandclinic.org

- Mayo Clinic Sexual Health Information:

    www.mayoclinic.org

Comprehensive Medical Resources:
- •MedlinePlus Erectile Dysfunction Guide:

    medlineplus.goverectiledysfunction.html
- •WebMD Erectile Dysfunction Health Center:

    www.webmd.com/erectile-dysfunction
- •NHS (UK) Erectile Dysfunction Information:

    www.nhs.uk/conditions/erection-problems-erectile-dysfunction

Support for Partners

These resources specifically address what you're going through as a partner. I wish we'd found some of these earlier, they would have saved us months of feeling like we were figuring everything out alone.

Partner-Specific Resources:
- •Coloplast Men's Health - Supporting a Partner with ED: www.coloplastmenshealth.com
- •Harvard Health - 7 Strategies for Partnering with ED: www.health.harvard.edu
- •WebMD ED Coping Guide:

www.webmd.com/erectile-dysfunction/erectile-dysfunction-coping

Online Communities and Forums:

Finding other people who understood what we were going through made a huge difference. These communities can provide support when you need to talk to someone who really gets it.

- Drugs.com ED Support Group: www.drugs.com/answers/support-group/erectile-dysfunction
- Reddit communities: r/DeadBedrooms, r/sexover30 (search for ED-related discussions)
- HealthUnlocked sexual health communities

Professional Help and Therapy

Sometimes you need more support than you can give each other. There's no shame in getting professional help, it shows how committed you are to working through this together.

Finding Therapists:

- American Association of Sexuality Educators, Counselors and Therapists (AASECT):

  www.aasect.org

- Psychology Today Therapist Directory:

  www.psychologytoday.com

- American Association for Marriage and Family Therapy: www.aamft.org

Specialized ED Support Groups:

- SoulUp ED Support Group (online): www.soulup.in
- Sexual Dysfunction Association (UK): www.sda.uk.net
- Local hospital-based support groups (contact urology departments)

Relationship and Sex Therapy:

If communication becomes difficult or you're feeling stuck, these organizations can help you find qualified therapists who understand sexual health challenges.

- Gottman Institute (relationship counseling):

    www.gottman.com
- Relate (UK relationship counseling):

    www.relate.org.uk
- International Society for Sexual Medicine:

    www.issm.info

Mental Health Support

ED can trigger depression and anxiety for both partners. Don't wait until things get overwhelming, these resources can provide support when you need it most.

General Mental Health:

- National Alliance on Mental Illness (NAMI):

    www.nami.org
- Depression and Bipolar Support Alliance:

    www.dbsalliance.org
- Anxiety and Depression Association of America:

    www.adaa.org

Crisis Support:

If either of you are struggling with thoughts of self-harm, please reach out immediately. These services are available 24/7.

- National Suicide Prevention Lifeline: 988
- Crisis Text Line: Text HOME to 741741
- SAMHSA National Helpline: 1-800-662-4357

Lifestyle and Health Resources

We learned that overall health impacts sexual function significantly. These resources helped us understand how diet, exercise, and general wellness connect to ED treatment.

Diet and Nutrition:

- •Academy of Nutrition and Dietetics:

  www.eatright.org

- •American Heart Association (heart-healthy diet):

  www.heart.org

Exercise and Physical Health:

- •Physical Activity Guidelines for Americans:

  health.gov/paguidelines

- •American Diabetes Association: www.diabetes.org

Books for Further Reading

Reading helped us both understand what we were experiencing and gave us new ways to talk about difficult topics. These books come from my personal recommendations and those of other couples I've spoken with.

For Partners:

- •"Come As You Are" by Emily Nagoski

- •"Mating in Captivity" by Esther Perel

- •"The Seven Principles for Making Marriage Work" by John Gottman ("A Summary of the 7 Principles for Making Marriage Work")

About Sexual Health:

- •"The Sexual Male" by Barry McCarthy and Michael Metz
- •"Mind Over Mood" by Dennis Greenberger and Christine Padesky
- •"Getting the Sex You Want" by Tammy Nelson

Communication and Relationships:

- •"Hold Me Tight" by Sue Johnson
- •"Attached" by Amir Levine and Rachel Heller
- •"The Five Love Languages" by Gary Chapman

Specialized Medical Resources

If ED is connected to other health conditions, these organizations provide condition-specific information that can help you understand the bigger picture.

For Specific Conditions:

- •American Diabetes Association: www.diabetes.org (diabetes-related ED)
- •American Heart Association: www.heart.org (cardiovascular-related ED)
- •American Cancer Society: www.cancer.org

  (cancer treatment-related ED)

Hormone-Related Resources:

- •Endocrine Society: www.endocrine.org
- •American Association of Clinical Endocrinologists: www.aace.com

Online Education and Support

Many hospitals and medical organizations offer free educational programs. Don't overlook these, we learned a lot from webinars that helped us ask better questions during medical appointments.

Webinars and Online Programs:

- •Many hospitals offer free online seminars about ED.
- •AASECT offers online continuing education (some open to public)
- •Check with local medical centers for patient education programs.

Reliable Health Websites:

When you're researching online, stick to these established medical sites. They provide accurate information without the sensationalism you'll find elsewhere.

- •Healthline: www.healthline.com
- •Verywell Health: www.verywellhealth.com
- •Medical News Today: www.medicalnewstoday.com

A Final Note on Research

I know the temptation to research everything but try not to overwhelm yourself. Pick one or two resources that feel most relevant to where you are right now. You can always come back to this list when you're ready for more information.

Always verify that any online resource is current and from a reputable medical organization. When in doubt, ask your healthcare provider about the reliability of information sources. Your doctor can help you sort through conflicting information and focus on what's most relevant to your specific situation.

For additional resources and updates:

www.jayrichard.com

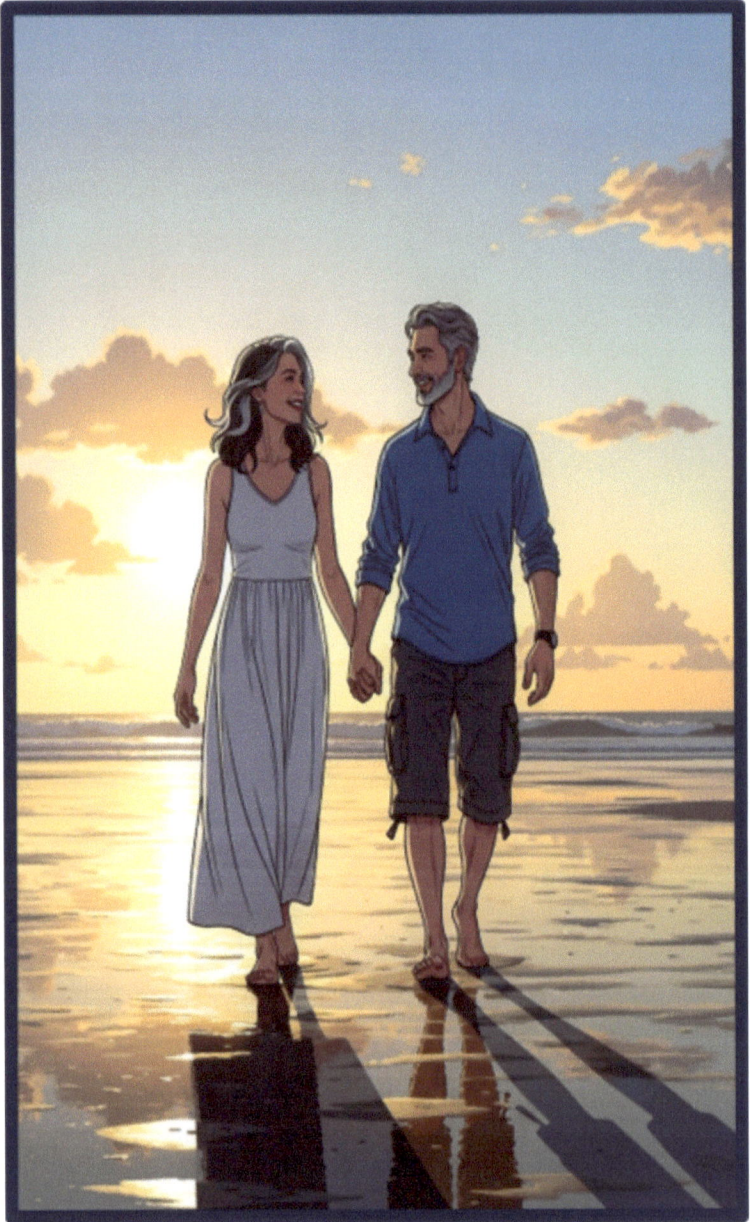

When Hope Is Found!

www.ingramcontent.com/pod-product-compliance
Lightning Source LLC
Chambersburg PA
CBHW040937030426
42335CB00001B/19